Beyond Avogadro's Number

Hahnemann's Private Battle which
Lead to the Discovery of Homeopathy

by

Allan Bonsall

B. Jain Publishers (P) Ltd.
An ISO 9001 : 2000 Certified Company
USA—EUROPE—INDIA

BEYOND AVOGADRO'S NUMBER

First Edition: 2009
1st Impression: 2009

All rights reserved. No part of this book may be reproduced, stored in a retrieval system or transmitted, in any form or by any means, mechanical, photocopying, recording or otherwise, without any prior written permission of the author.

© with the author

Published by Kuldeep Jain for
B. JAIN PUBLISHERS (P) LTD.
An ISO 9001 : 2000 Certified Company
1921/10, Chuna Mandi, Paharganj, New Delhi 110 055 (INDIA)
Tel.: 91-11-2358 0800, 2358 1100, 2358 1300, 2358 3100
Fax: 91-11-2358 0471 • *Email:* info@bjain.com
Website: **www.bjainbooks.com**

Printed in India by
J.J. Offset Printers

ISBN: 978-81-319-0742-9

Foreword

Homeopathy has gained the reputation as the most popular complementary system of medicine of today. Ever since its principles were codified by Dr. Christian Friedrich Samuel Hahnemann of Germany, some of its unconventional approaches continue to be a mystery to the material scientists. Known for his critical views on the existing medical paradigm, Hahnemann was ahead of his time in postulating concepts, theories and principles for a new medical system based on the unexplored concepts of Hippocrates, the father of medicine and ancient medical scriptures. Hahnemann was less concerned that his theories and principles stood the test of his time, than he was with the safety, efficacy and scientificity of medicine. Thus he gifted a humane system of medicine to mankind. The modern medical world is indebted to him for being the reformer of the barbaric practice of the old medical thoughts.

For the critics of his system, Homeopathy is a saga; for the patients who receive its benefits Homeopathy is a panacea, and for its practitioners, Homeopathy is a mission. Some of the concepts and theories of Hahnemann continue to intrigue the world. However, the acceptance of the system is ever growing for the health care needs of the public. After all, none of the medical systems being practiced today could explain everything which occurs in the system. Medicine has been an odyssey ever since it got organized.

The life of Samuel Hahnemann, the man credited with creating the medical philosophy of homeopathy, is well documented. Equally well documented is his ambitious struggle to bring his system of medicine into being. *Beyond Avogadro's Number* by Allan Bonsall tells the story of Samuel Hahnemann's fight with the physicians of the old school and the apothecaries who held royal monopolies over the making and dispensing of medicines. It talks of Hahnemann's private battle which lead to the discovery of Homeopathy.

It is difficult to feel comfortable in defining this story as fiction because so much of it is based on fact. But it cannot be classified a biography of the life of Samuel Hahnemann because the story deliberately, and without apology, introduces fictitious characters and unproven events. To call it a "biopic", which seems to be the favoured term of the moviemakers, conjures a sense of commercialisation that is so out of keeping with the principles of the man that it cannot be used without all loss of credibility.

Neither is it a story about homeopathy. Perhaps the book can best be described as a fictionalized biography. It endeavors to tell the story of Hahnemann's fight with the apothecaries in such a way that brings it to life. It is the story of one man's fight against the established code, a code that existed not because it was proven right but because it had the luxury of historical precedent.

As the author has rightly put it, "the more one reads about Hahnemann, the more one becomes intrigued by his fight to establish his modality", Homeopathy can be understood only through deeper study and understanding of its philosophical concepts. Looking at it from the shadows and pointing fingers only perpetuates the myths. Professionalism shall come only from consistency and endeavor to swim into its deeper water.

Allan Bonsall is not a scientific author. His style of presenting the book is to entertain, and seeks to bring the characters to life. However, the work is more important for the reason that it was seen and corrected by the great Homeopathic historian Dr. Julian Winston towards the end of his life.

Dr. Eswara Das

Acknowledgements

The writing of *Beyond Avogadro's Number* had a unique genesis and cannot be allowed to pass without acknowledging the people who inspired me to even attempt it.

At the outset I have to confess that my own demons drew me to homeopathy. For the better part of three decades I worked in the high pressure business of advertising, climbing, for better or worse, to the top of the corporate ladder. For most of those years I struggled with depression, finding little, if any, help in either the drugs or the psychiatry that was offered. In the end, that struggle cost me a career, a marriage and nearly my health. I say nearly because, although my career and my marriage were gone, my health was saved by homeopathy.

Without doubt the catalyst to my writing *Beyond Avogadro's Number* was George Christinson. George is Principal of the Academy of Homeopathic Medicine in Brisbane and the healer who brought me blessed relief from what was going on inside my head. Unbeknownst to me, Elizabeth Wighton, a student at the Academy and owner of an on-line bookshop *Similibooks*, had just donated a range of books on Samuel Hahnemann to the Academy's library. It was from these resources that I was able to piece together those parts of Hahnemann's story that emerge through the telling of this tale.

Since that beginning, Elizabeth and George have been towers of confidence whenever the demons looked set to return.

Another homeopath played a key role. Glenis Black and her husband, Peter, are old friends. Glenis has recently graduated as a homeopath. Whilst she was studying, Peter and I often indulged ourselves in the less rigorous pastime of tennis. On one such occasion I tore a muscle in my left quad. The injury kept me away from the courts for nearly a month, and when I finally returned it was only to have the damage recur. This time Peter was having nothing to do with my intentions to seek medical help and insisted that we go to his home for coffee, and a free consultation with Glen.

I'm still not sure what homeopathic remedy Glen gave me, but half an hour later the pain had gone and I was walking comfortably. The next weekend I was playing tennis without any discomfort. As far as homeopathy was concerned, I was hooked, and the more I read about Hahnemann, the more I became intrigued by his fight to establish his modality.

It was also Glenis Black who saw the potential in the name for the book, ringing me early one morning with the suggestion of *Beyond Avogadro's Number*.

Homeopathy often requires people to demonstrate a considerable leap of faith. The critics point to the dilution of remedies, specifically that when a substance has been diluted a thousand times it cannot possibly contain any of the original matter. In the early 1800s Amadeo Avogadro calculated a value, what has since become known as Avogadro's Number or Constant, for the number of atoms or molecules in a gram mole of any substance. A "mole" is defined in the International System of Units (SI) as Avogadro's number of particles of any kind of substance.

I refer to Avogadro's number in the book and was taken to task on this point by the late Julian Winston, esteemed historian, author and homeopath (not to mention slide guitarist), for referring to Avogadro at a time when, historically, Hahnemann may not have heard or known of the theory. I checked my facts and discovered that Avogadro's number came into being in 1811, whilst my reference in the book took place after 1813.

I met Julian only a few months before his sad passing. It was at a Slide Guitar Music Festival in Brisbane, and Elizabeth Wighton took me along to meet him. After he had played, and I must acknowledge he did so with a style and energy that left many of his compatriots in his shadow, we met and discussed my manuscript. Reluctantly he agreed to read it, reluctantly because he had been burned before by sensationalised and badly-written attempts to do something similar. At this time, Julian's fight with the cancer that would ultimately take his life had begun to take its toll, yet I received his response in a long email only a few weeks later. His opening remarks, I'm assured, were rare praise indeed, but he tempered his comments by pointing out some of the classic blunders I had made. Given that now they are, in the main, corrected, I think I can be excused from going into too much detail.

What Julian said by way of praise, and his detailed comments about the historical facts of the manuscript, were a great fillip and gave me the confidence to take this to the next step. To that end it would be remiss of me not to thank Stephen Thompson, editor extraordinaire, and the man who pushed the right buttons to get this thing published. As an outcome, if I can encourage one person to trial homeopathy for their own well-being then the effort will have been worthwhile.

And finally, to my dearest Jann, without whose support this journey would never have begun.

Publisher's Note

We all who are reading this book are connected to homeopathy in some way and are therefore indebted to the man who gave birth to this science, Dr. Christian Friedrich Samuel Hahnemann. Most of the students or followers of homeopathy have read the life history of Dr. Hahnemann in their initial years of study but what we all remember at the end of the day is the Linehour Barla experiment & the origin of homeopathy. Its said you have to know your history to cast a future for yourself. The author has given a totally new dimension to the life history of Hahnemann by depicting the facts in a new way and all the circumstances have been so beautifully written that you feel as if you are watching it happen in front of your eyes. The story does involve some fictitious characters at certain places to fill in the gaps. It gives us an idea of what circumstances led Hahnemann to look out for a new system of healing altogether. Today, when everybody is trying their hands at fiction and we all love to read a novel, this homeopathic story is one such which I recommend to all homeopaths to read atleast once & see or rather feel the drama of homeopathy.

Kuldeep Jain
C.E.O., B. Jain Publisher's (P) Ltd.

Contents

Foreword .... *iii*
Acknowledgements .... *v*
Publisher's note .... *ix*

PART ONE
Saxony 1791–1793 1

PART TWO
Saxony 1793 – 1794 59

PART THREE
Konigslutter, 1799 109

PART FOUR
Leipzig, 1811 – 1813 145

PART FIVE
Leipzig, 1816 – 1817 211

PART SIX
Leipzig, 1819 – 1821 273
Postscript 351

PART ONE

SAXONY 1791 – 1793

1

The black stallion stood five and a half feet at the shoulder, its flanks glistening from the passing rainsquall. Steam poured from the magnificent beast's flared nostrils, its teeth bared against the silver of the bridle, foam and spittle edging the bit.

Samuel moved the curtain to gain a clearer view of the swayed-back bridge forty yards away. He'd expected the arrogance and power of the horse to be reflected in the eyes of its rider and wasn't disappointed. Even in the darkening sky the cavalry officer's eyes flashed white under his black leather helmet and proud black comb.

The officer turned in the saddle to face back the way he had come. Misty rain curled across the greatcoat that draped unbuttoned from his wide shoulders. Samuel could see the white double-breasted *kollet* the cuirassiers wore into battle, spurning the protection of armour for speed. A white leather shoulder strap bisected the double row of brass buttons on the tunic. At the cuirassier's throat, the poppy red of his collar was the only other concession to the military drabness of black and grey. After a brief moment the officer returned his gaze to the front, his eyes narrowing as he searched the road ahead.

A stifled moan dragged Samuel from the window. Four

young children were huddled in the corner of the room. The eldest, a girl no more than eight, held a sleeping toddler in her arms. A crude curtain separated the children from the source of the cry.

'She will be here soon, my sweet Elise, have courage.' Even as the words left Samuel Hahnemann's mouth something told him the midwife would be too frightened to come on such a night.

His wife searched his face for the lie. Squaring his shoulders, Samuel returned her gaze with piercing eyes that accentuated his aquiline features. At thirty-six he felt stronger than he had as a boy, perhaps more so than he had even as a young man, and yet sometime in the past few years his hair had turned from fair to white. Of even greater chagrin was that he had lost much of it, revealing a strong forehead.

He crossed to the bed and clasped his wife's hand, feeling the gathering urgency of her labour. With his free hand he picked up the damp cloth from the small table beside the bed.

'It is a godless eve, Elise, and there are strange riders about. The midwife may be forced to wait until the streets are clear,' Samuel said, wiping his wife's brow with the tepid cloth. He made a mental note to check the kettle on the small stove.

A noise of approaching thunder slowly grew, until a low steady boom filled the room. Samuel rushed to the window, glimpsing from the corner of his eye the frightened faces of his children. The toddler had woken, unsure of where the noise had come from, not knowing whether to cry from fear or for attention. Outside, the noise mimicked the sound of rain lashing the roof, only amplified a hundred times. He nervously flicked the curtain to one side and peered through the grimy glass pane. In the deepening gloom he could just make out the flashing legs of cavalry horses pounding along the cobbled street. Samuel's heart skipped a beat as a different noise rose above the pounding hooves. He strained his ears to identify the new sound.

Samuel left the window and flung the door open. The steaming flank of a horse filled his view, the same black beauty he had seen on the bridge only minutes before.

His nose was only inches from the officer's grey clad legs. He could smell the dampness on the red saddlecloth. Above him the Prussian officer paid Samuel no heed, oblivious to the light spilling through the partially open door as his men streamed past.

Samuel cleared his throat, the sound consumed in the bedlam around him. 'Why is the Prussian cavalry crossing through Saxony?' he yelled.

The cuirassier raised himself in the stirrups to peer over his shoulder, the new sound swelling, adding to the noise of tramping hooves. Finally the officer lowered himself back into his saddle and peered down at Samuel, a look of disdain on his face.

'We travel on the king's business, with the blessing of Frederick Augustus.'

'W ...what business possibly needs this kind of army?' Samuel asked, intimidated by the man's air. He could now see the troop of grey clad infantrymen pouring over the swayed-back bridge. At the head of the troop a dozen drummers gave the men their marching beat.

'The fools in France,' yelled the major, his rank now visible. 'The fools who threaten to cut off their King's head.'

'But why are you marching against the French revolutionaries? They haven't invaded us. Why would they want to?'

'I follow my orders and mind my business. You would be advised to mind yours.'

Without another word the major pushed his boots into the side of the stallion. The horse reared briefly before moving off beside the body of infantry that now filled the road from culvert to culvert and to well beyond the bridge.

Samuel returned inside closing the door with his rump. He leaned against it, his head spinning with the major's revelation.

So Saxony had once again thrown its lot in with their powerful neighbour.

An anguished cry from his wife broke into his thoughts.

'I am sorry, Elise. The roads are choked with soldiers, it will be impossible for the midwife to get here. Unfortunately you will have to allow my help.' Samuel smiled at his wife, Johanna Henriette Hahnemann, his beloved Elise, the only endearment she truly loved to hear him use.

He crossed to the small hearth and picked up the kettle. Steam leaked from the metal spout. He smiled across at the children to reassure them, the eldest girl, and a boy a year younger, returned his smile with uncertain efforts of their own. Later, Samuel thought to himself, I will explain everything to them.

He joined his wife behind the curtain just as her face contorted in a grimace of pain. He smiled gently as Johanna opened her eyes.

'Do not feel embarrassed that your husband should be here. In some ways I am better trained than the midwife.' He raised his brow. 'My medical degree should surely count for something,' Samuel teased his wife.

'What ...?' Johanna paused to catch her breath. 'What is happening, Samuel Hahnemann? What disaster besets us now?' Another contraction whipped her breath away.

Samuel poured the contents of the kettle into the bowl, picked up a cloth and dipped it in the hot water. 'It seems that our good Prince Frederick has thrown his lot in with the Prussians.' Samuel gathered the towels laid out in preparation for the midwife. 'They are on their way to protect our borders from the French.' His eyebrows lifted. 'I had thought they were too busy taking each other's heads to worry about us. Two days ago the news was that King Louis had acquiesced to the demands of the republicans who now rule the parliament in Paris ...' Samuel paused as Johanna's body trembled with another spasm. 'How far apart are they?'

Johanna gasped as she fought to keep her breathing under control. 'I counted to sixty that time. I think our newest daughter is very impatient to join us.'

'Our daughter? You are so sure that the baby is a girl?'

Her reply came through gritted teeth. 'Oh I am sure, Doctor Hahnemann. I am very sure.'

2

The candle flickered at his elbow casting a soft glow across the papers and books littering the small kitchen table. Samuel stared at the words on the page of the massive tome, the fingers of his left hand sliding uncertainly from side to side searching for the words he had lost. With the quill, he scratched at a persistent itch high on his forehead. The curtain moved. He ignored it, dipped the quill into the ink and carefully added an annotation to the page that was already covered in his flowing script.

'Have you not laboured enough for one night?' Johanna whispered softly as she gently pulled the curtain to one side. Her hair hung loose from her sleep, her eyes still half closed. 'The children will be waking soon; you should try to get some sleep.' She slipped past the curtain, a knitted shawl pulled over her flannel nightdress, a simple bow on the bodice the only concession to style.

'Another hour, Elise,' Samuel whispered. 'I have nearly finished one of the most difficult and intricate chapters. Cullen's work is brilliant, but there are times when I think he has missed the most basic point.' Samuel shrugged his shoulders. 'What can we expect of a man who writes in English, the most convoluted of languages, and a Scotsman to boot.'

Samuel didn't wait to see if his wife appreciated his humour, turning instead back to the sheet of writing paper to complete the annotation he had started. Johanna stood at his shoulder admiring the neat, flowing script. As she read, her smile disappeared, replaced by a thin line of displeasure.

'Oh no, Samuel. Please promise me you are not going to start experimenting on yourself again.' Her whisper was more strident than that of a moment before. 'This is impossible. We barely have enough to live on without you turning from your translation work.'

'Hush, Elise.' Samuel laid the quill next to the small stand holding the inkwell and turned to take his wife's hand. 'I know it is not easy for you and the children, especially now that there are seven of us. For the moment I do not intend to resume my provings, but that does not turn me from my thoughts or my beliefs. This man Cullen,' Samuel pointed to the massive volume opened on the table, 'claims that cinchona works because of its tonic effect on the stomach. That it cured the Vice Queen of Peru, no less. The Vice Queen, whatever that means.'

'Please, Samuel, keep your voice down.'

Samuel pushed his chair back, maintaining his hold on Johanna's hand. He lowered his voice until it was barely above a whisper. 'Peruvian bark works because it can produce symptoms similar to those of intermittent fever in healthy people. I proved that through my experiment on myself. When I took just four drams of the damned substance twice a day, my feet and fingertips became cold. Then I became languid and drowsy. You remember, Elise? You saw me go through it.' Samuel watched his wife nod, the look on her face subdued, patient.

'It was frightening, and it was tempering at the same time,' Samuel continued. 'When my heart began to palpitate and my pulse to race, an intolerable anxiety and trembling took over my very being. Remember how ill I became?' He squeezed her hand unaware of her exaggerated patience. 'All the symptoms of intermittent fever, including redness of my cheeks, unquenchable thirst, pounding headaches, all of them laid me low until I stopped taking the medicine. Yet this noble Scotsman ...' Samuel punched a condescending finger towards the volume on his table, ' ... would have us believe that cinchona acts as a trifling tonic on the stomach. When will these doctors learn?'

Samuel Hahnemann slipped his hand from his wife's and reached across the table to pick up the quill, his demeanour calm again. 'Another hour will see the chapter finished then I will help you with the children. Perhaps later I can take Henrietta and Friedrich for a walk in the fresh air. It will do us all a world of good.'

Samuel watched Henrietta and Friedrich playing beside the stream. A hundred yards away he could see the small swayed-back bridge where the Prussian major had waited for his cavalry troop and infantry. Spreading out from both sides of the bridge were the backs of the houses that lined the main street of Stotteritz. He smiled, recalling the mortified look on the face of his beloved Elise when he'd told her the midwife would be unlikely to risk coming out on such a night.

He wondered briefly about the fate of the Prussian major. Talk in the town had been full of the revolution and turmoil in France. It had been the only topic of discussion around the apothecary and the inn for days. The rumours had grown wilder and wilder, reaching their climax with reports that tens of thousands of French men and women had been slaughtered simply because they were suspected of opposing Robespierre. Finally, word had come to confirm the Prussian major's words. Emboldened by their success the revolutionary army had sought other spoils and were striking out against their neighbours to take revenge on those who had given succour to the fleeing aristocracy. The allied Prussian and Saxon armies had fought hard to turn back the French revolutionaries from the German border, with many men killed on both sides.

The smile slipped from Samuel's face as he imagined the horror. He shook his head in a silent prayer. *Why, oh why do people so needlessly waste each other's lives?*

Samuel climbed to his feet. He brushed the grass from his woollen pants, reached down to straighten the short hose on his legs and caught a glimpse of the scuffed toes of his black pumps.

'Friedrich, Henrietta, quickly,' Samuel called out. 'I must go to the pharmacy. I need to speak to the apothecary to see if some supplies I ordered have arrived.' Samuel picked up the woollen topcoat he'd left lying on the grass. Slipping his arms into the sleeves, he smiled self-consciously at the leather patches Johanna had sewn on to cover the thinning cloth at the left elbow.

The two children rushed to his side, colour bursting from their cheeks, and, together, the three walked across the field to a small laneway that allowed them access to the road.

Passing their lodgings, Samuel inclined his head, half expecting to see Johanna and the other three children sunning themselves on the front steps. There was no-one there; the front door was closed. Perhaps, he thought, she has taken the children for a short walk to the butcher. He had received a small stipend from the publishers in Leipzig, and Johanna had promised to treat them to some sausage.

Friedrich dawdled at the small bridge, his attention taken by the flash of sun on the water. Henrietta chattered away to her father, her small hand sneaking into his. Samuel smiled down into the laughing eyes of his eldest daughter, his favourite, although it was not an admission he would make publicly. Behind them, tired of the small stream, Freidrich looked up to make sure his father and sister were not too far away. Smiling, he waved then jumped to his feet and ran hard to catch up to them. As he came level, he grabbed for his father's free hand, giving his sister a haughty look. Samuel laughed at the antics of the boy. Soon they were all laughing, his daughter loudest of all.

'I see that your youngsters are in good health, Doctor Hahnemann. Perhaps the country food agrees with them?'

Samuel looked up from his laughing children, recognising the voice of Albert Wagner. The local apothecary towered above him by three or four inches, his dark hair curling at the sides and back of his head. He wore a topcoat of the finest wool tailored in Leipzig to hide his rapidly increasing girth. Around his neck was wrapped a scarf of the finest imported silk.

Behind the apothecary a group of the town's menfolk had gathered to enjoy the early spring warmth and to discuss the news of the day.

Samuel nodded to Wagner and then turned to acknowledge the other men, their response subdued. Samuel kept his face passive, well aware of the rumours about the doctor who had forsaken the practice of his craft for the writing of books. He was not writing them, he had tried to say, he was translating them. How were the more enlightened of his fellow doctors to learn the skills being forged elsewhere unless someone troubled themselves to translate the new theories from the English or the Greek, or even the Latin in which they were written? Typical, he thought, of the ignorance of many of his countrymen. They had their heads buried in sand, just like so many of the doctors of his birth land.

'I trust you are well, Herr Wagner,' Samuel replied. 'I have come to see if the chemicals I ordered have arrived.'

The apothecary nodded, his expression giving nothing away, his eyes not leaving Hahnemann's. 'Yes, they came in this morning on the coach with my own supplies.' He continued to coldly appraise Samuel before finally breaking the spell, clearly irritated by the two children waiting quietly and patiently at Hahnemann's side, so unlike the unruly behaviour of his own three youngsters. His annoyance surfaced openly as he looked into the clear eyes of the doctor. 'I hope it is not your intention to start preparing and dispensing your own medicines?'

Slowly Samuel shook his head, caution making him refrain from a more blunt response. His eyes held Wagner's, refusing to back down. 'They are for simple chemical experiments to help with my translations. I have no current desire to either practice or prescribe, I can assure you.'

Wagner nodded. 'Just as well. I'm sure I don't have to remind you of the laws.'

With his rightful position restored in front of the other men, the apothecary tempered his superior air, the arrogance slipping from his eyes. Samuel wondered if the conversation would now follow its predictable course.

'How is your wife, Herr doctor? Well, I hope,' Wagner asked, his tone still abrupt.

'Thank you, she is very well.' Samuel peered guilelessly at Wagner. *Damn him for his hypocrisy*, he railed inside before continuing quietly. 'The new baby is now eight months old and well settled. Her grandfather would have been very proud of her,' Samuel added deliberately, knowing full well that Wagner's question had been prompted by the standing of Johanna's late father, who had been an influential apothecary in Dessau.

Wagner turned on his heel. 'I will get you the parcel. There was also a letter delivered by the coachman.'

Samuel willed himself to remain patient. Beside him his children stood quietly, their eyes fixed on the ground, while the men at the apothecary shifted uncomfortably.

He had made no attempt to become acquainted with any of them and was contemptuous of their fawning relationship with Wagner. Yet the tradition was long standing. Business was conducted at these daily gatherings, and newcomers were introduced to other established businessmen of the town. Ten years ago Samuel would have eagerly availed himself of the tradition, knowing that a young doctor would be stupid to try and establish a practice without the blessing of the local pharmacy.

The men fell into a desultory conversation about the fortunes of the French. Conjecture abounded on the likelihood of their prince following in his father's footsteps by changing sides. A chuckle broke from one of the men, followed by a sly glance at Samuel, who kept his eyes glued on the doorway, angrily willing Wagner to return. Finally Wagner emerged, his arms filled with a sizeable parcel wrapped in paper and tied off with light twine. In the apothecary's pocket, Samuel spied a large buff envelope.

Grateful to be nearing the end of this charade, Samuel

adopted a more conciliatory tone. 'Thank you for your trouble, Herr Wagner. Do I owe you anything?'

Wagner shook his head, also happy to see the business to an end. 'No,' he blustered. 'No, it is my duty. The bill for the chemicals has been added to your account. Perhaps you could settle the outstanding amount next time you are in the shop.'

Samuel burned at the insinuation, having settled his account only a few days before. He nodded brusquely, paying no attention to the assembled smirks and grins of the chattering men. He turned and left, his two children trotting happily behind unaware of their father's anger, the letter clutched tightly in Henrietta's hand.

Samuel's eyes were fixed on the wax seal. The envelope was of the finest parchment, his name written in the most beautiful hand on the front.

'Samuel, please open the letter,' Johanna pleaded. 'You can't sit there all day just staring at it.'

'The arrogance of the man,' he blurted out. 'How dare he infer that I had not paid his bill. They are convinced that they own the world.' He shook his head. 'No, that's not it at all. No, they're convinced the world owes them a living. How dare he?'

'Oh, for goodness sake.' Johanna reached out a hand. 'Give the letter to me. If it is bad news, best that we know the extent of it.' Trying to lighten the mood, she smiled at her husband. 'Perhaps it is an offer of a job,' she said. 'Perhaps he's writing to offer you the job as personal doctor to the duke.' Johanna had also seen the seal and knew of the reputation of Duke Ernst of Saxe-Coburg-Gotha.

Samuel tore his eyes away from the envelope to look at his wife. 'What?' he said, his anger blotting out everything Johanna had said.

'Nothing,' Johanna said crossly. 'Give me the letter. If you don't intend to open it I will.'

Samuel looked at the letter in his hands then flipped it onto the table, his anger unabated. 'It is probably a criticism of my last newspaper article.'

'Samuel, please. Your paranoia about the apothecaries will make your brain explode. You forget that my late father was a man of this noble calling, and my stepfather also. They are both honourable men, at least my father was when he was alive, and I will not have you impugn the reputations of all apothecaries simply because Herr Wagner has insulted you. I swear there are days ...' Johanna threw her hands up in the air. 'Oh, this is ridiculous. Open the letter before I say something the children shouldn't hear.'

'You know perfectly well how highly I regarded your father,' Samuel replied. 'This is not an argument about honourable men; this is about the power the apothecaries wield, and the arrogant way that most of them use it. As for your stepfather...' Samuel looked up. Johanna stood over him, her hands on her hips. Any vestige of patience had fled her face, her eyes narrowed, daring her husband to continue.

Without another word Samuel picked up the letter from where it lay. Gingerly he slid a paperknife through the seal. He scanned down the page, not stopping until he had reached the end.

'Well, Samuel, is it from the duke personally?' Johanna asked, her anger forgotten.

Samuel looked up from the letter blind to the excitement on his wife's face.

'Please, Samuel. Now you are being cruel to all of us.'

He took in the rest of his dismal surroundings, seeing the children gathered around their mother's skirts, the baby gurgling contentedly in the arms of his eldest daughter, the second youngest happily playing on the floor beside her siblings.

'Samuel, I insist,' Johanna stamped her foot in frustration, 'what does the duke say?'

Samuel dropped his eyes once more to the letter. He re-read the first few lines before replying, his words stuttering at the start. 'You were right. He has offered me a job. The duke has offered me a job,' he repeated, the wonder in his voice hard to disguise.

'What, as his personal physician? As the house's doctor?' Johanna's eyes flew around the single room. Perhaps, she dared hope ... perhaps?

Slowly Samuel shook his head, his eyes flicking to the page again before handing the letter across.

'No, not as his physician. Not even as a doctor in Gotha. The duke wants me to run an asylum. An insane asylum in Georgenthal.'

3

'It still intrigues me, my good doctor, what brought you to write the article in the first place?'

Samuel peered at the Duke of Gotha. 'I'm sorry your grace, it has been a long and tiring journey and I still don't think I have my wits fully about me. But I, er, I must point out that the editor of *Der Anzeiger*, Councillor Becker, put his own name to the article.'

'Come now, my good doctor. Let's not begin our friendship on a lie. Herr Becker is not only a good friend of yours, he is also a good friend of mine.' The duke shook his head, smiling indulgently as he lumbered to his feet.

He was a large man, well into his middle years and still fit from his hunting, although he favoured his right leg. 'Please excuse my apparent inconvenience.' A rueful grin spread across his face. 'I fell from my mount this morning when it became excited by the first deer of the season.' Beside him the fire burned heartily, the fresh scent of newly cut logs pleasantly pervading the room. Spring had well and truly arrived, but the warmth of the days still struggled to keep the cold away from the mountains as evening fell. His hand engulfed the small bell resting on the mantle above the hearth. Almost immediately a liveried servant appeared at the door.

'Some refreshment, Doctor Hahnemann, I understand you are partial to a light beer.'

'Thank you, your grace, a beer would be welcome. I am somewhat parched.'

The duke nodded at the servant. 'I think I will enjoy some of the whisky our last guests brought.'

The servant bowed briefly and left. The duke busied himself with the fire before turning back to his guest. 'I am sure you will find Georgenthal a beautiful place.'

'I have no doubt, your grace. Please, forgive my rudeness. Yes, I did write the article you refer to, but asked Herr Becker to put it under his name lest my detractors saw fit to bombard the paper with letters attacking me rather than the thoughts expressed.'

'Is that not somewhat self-indulgent, my friend?' The duke's eyebrows rose a fraction.

'Perhaps, but accurate, I can assure you. I think too many of the good doctors of Saxony have either too much time on their hands or are fearful that their barbarous practices will be spurned by their unsuspecting patients and they will lose their livelihood.' Samuel's eyes had narrowed to slits, his efforts at being civil on the subject sorely testing him. 'The article would have been seen as no different to my previous attack on their more damning practice of venesection. There is no question that their bloodletting caused the death of Emperor Leopold.'

'Please, my good doctor, please calm yourself,' the duke said, surprised at the sudden passion in his guest's voice.

The servant appeared carrying a silver salver. On the tray stood a tankard of beer and a crystal glass half filled with whisky. Beside the tumbler sat a small glass jug of water.

'Ah, refreshments,' the duke said, grateful for the intrusion. The servant placed the tankard on a small table beside Samuel. The duke took the moment to digest the surprising measure of dislike Hahnemann had for his fellow doctors. 'Enjoy, my friend,' the duke said, tipping a dash of water into his glass and raising it to his guest. 'Here's to your continuing good health.'

'And to you, your grace, for your kind hospitality.'

The duke smiled over the rim of his glass. 'Oh, I have no doubt that you will earn your board and keep, as well as the fees you propose to charge your patients. But, please, continue. Do you seriously believe that people will accept you can cure the insane?'

'It will take time,' Samuel said, 'but ultimately, yes, I do, your grace. These patients are ill, mentally ill, but they are treated like wild animals. Our institutions chain them and beat them and put them on public display for the amusement of the people. There is no respect for them as human beings so they simply become objects of abuse.' Samuel suppressed a yawn, shuddering at the images in his mind.

The duke remained silent, equally well-versed in the apparent hopelessness of the insane. His lips pursed tightly in agreement. He lifted his drink, but spoke before taking a sip. 'It has been a long day for you, my friend, perhaps you should rest. We can resume our discussions tomorrow when you have slept.'

'I'm sorry, your grace, you must think me a hopeless case. Yes, I am tired, but I am also excited.' Samuel slapped his hands together, a light shining briefly in his eyes, 'For years I have been studying diseases of the most lingering and hopeless nature, and have long suspected that the mental is as important as the physical when it comes to understanding some of these ailments. I believe many diseases originate in the mind, or are significantly influenced by emotional causes. I am yet to provide overwhelming evidence but I am more and more of the opinion that emotional stress caused by anxiety and even exposure to fright is one of the most significant discoveries waiting for us to make.'

'But surely there are doctors who specialise in illnesses of the brain who apply their skills to the treatment of the insane?'

'Those with the right skills are few and far between. Frankly, I do not know of one doctor living today who I would entrust with my own health if I were to become ill from some malady of the brain.' Samuel paused. His hand briefly stroked the side of his face, 'With the exception of Pinel. But he resides in Paris, so that isn't an option.'

The duke shook his head, his jowls shaking. 'Surely, doctor, you jest. This is the eighteenth century, for goodness sake; we aren't living in the dark ages. There must be someone, some doctor in all of Saxony who you would trust?'

A great weight seemed to descend on Samuel. 'We have far too many doctors who believe the cause of disease lies in the blood, so they drain as much as they can. When their bloodletting fails, they assault the body with large doses of medicines, although they have no understanding of the possible side-effects.'

The duke remained impassive, his face carefully composed, his arms crossed.

Ignoring the silent censure, Samuel continued. 'If the doctors haven't already killed the patient, they resort to using palliatives that effectively mask the disease by opposing it; in essence, persuading the patient that they weren't sick in the first place. Then, if everything that has transpired to this point is not enough, the doctor invents a name for the malady, preferably one with Greek origins so that the patient is suitably impressed and deems that the doctor clearly must know what he is doing. That, I'm afraid, your grace is the sum total of the way our doctors work.'

The duke regarded Samuel gravely. 'I have read some of your work, Doctor Hahnemann. I respect much of what you have said and I think I have some understanding of your position, but I find it almost beyond belief that the entire medical fraternity does not have some redeeming position to offer.' He leant forward in his chair. 'If what you say carries any weight, then perhaps I should be pleased by my own acumen in offering you this post.' The duke paused to weigh up his words before continuing. 'Or perhaps I should be fearful of your arrogance and what you might do.'

For a moment Samuel hesitated, unsure how to reply. Clearly his host was a much more astute and sensitive man than most, but then that should not surprise him. Everything he knew about the duke had pointed to it. His compassion and charity had earned him accolades through the press as a true father of his people. Even the duke's invitation to take up this position came from his concern over the deplorable conditions many of his fellow nobles suffered in asylums.

'Your grace, I assure you that I will do everything in my power to bring health where there is sickness.' He paused to rally his thoughts. 'I can also assure you my pride shall have no bearing on that.'

Samuel got to his feet. 'Is our patient settled, your grace? I am eager to have the opportunity to meet him and begin his treatment.'

The duke followed, his leg causing him to grimace briefly. 'Herr Klockenbring is still to join us. He has been moved from Hanover and is currently interned in the asylum in Gotha. Tomorrow you should spend time settling into your new home. Then, if you feel up to it, I will arrange for you to return to Gotha and collect our guest. I cannot vouch for the condition in which you will find him. The last time I spoke with his good wife she was subdued. I am sure she is mortified by the conditions she finds her husband in whenever she visits. I will send word to the good lady that you have arrived. Perhaps you could spend some time with her in Gotha to reassure her of the good hands her husband is being delivered into, not to mention what treatment he will be receiving for her fees.'

4

'Elise, look at the sun filtering through those trees.' Samuel pointed across the small clearing, the toddler Amalie on his hip. 'Oh my beloved Saxony, this is why I love it so. Surely we are blessed to live in such a beautiful part of God's world, and how good is this air for the children?'

A short distance ahead, Henrietta squealed in delight. She pointed at the end of the clearing where a small doe bounded across the short gap. A loud crash followed as the doe's mother burst through the undergrowth. In one bound she crossed the path, chasing her newborn into the shrubs on the other side.

The children stood enthralled. A joyous whoop leapt from Friedrich.. His sister joined in until their father, also laughing, hushed them, warning them to be quiet if they wished to see more of the animals and the birds he had described to them over breakfast.

Quietly the family continued their walk through the sweeping forests and glades of the magnificent Thuringer Wald.

'Did you find the duke as you expected, Samuel? You were so tired when you returned to our rooms that I am sure you were asleep before your head touched the pillow. Even my most laboured shaking could not rouse you.' Johanna smiled.

'He is everything I had expected and been told, and then

some. Not only is he generous of spirit but is an articulate and clever man whose mind is open to new ideas. If I had any reason to question his intellect it could only be on his naiveté about the skills of our medical fraternity.'

'Will you have further opportunities to discuss your ideas with him?'

Samuel shook his head. 'Apparently he will be travelling with me to Gotha in the morning and intends to remain there. Perhaps he will return to his lodge to partake of the hunting, but he says he has a great deal of work to do in Gotha.'

'Did he give you any more insight into your first patient?' Johanna asked with a mischievous smile.

'Perhaps my *only* patient, Elise. As much as the announcement in Becker's paper suggested a nursing home for mental patients of the better classes, it appears there has been no interest shown by others of a similar indisposition. Or, perhaps I should say, shown by their families.'

'Surely dealing with only one patient will not be too onerous for someone as skilled as you,' Johanna teased.

'Your sarcasm is not as subtle as usual, my sweet Elise. Perhaps I should retract my earlier remarks?' Samuel regarded his wife, enjoying the smile on her ruddy cheeks. Her waist had thickened a little since they had married, but her pretty fresh face still softened his heart, the dark curls on her head mirroring the dark brown of her eyes that twinkled back at him.

'How did Herr Klockenbring come to the attention of the duke?'

'Apparently his wife saw the article I wrote and approached Herr Becker.'

'But I thought you had asked Herr Becker to keep your name from any association with those ideas,' Johanna said.

'Becker and the duke had often discussed my writings. My article appears to have been a catalyst for the duke to make his offer after hearing of the sufferings of Herr Klockenbring.'

'But why should Herr Klockenbring have caused the duke such personal concern? Wasn't he Minister of Police and

Secretary to the Chancellor of Hanover? Hanover is a long way from Gotha,' Johanna remarked.

'All I know is that Herr Klockenbring was a highly respected official who, for many years, has been afflicted with the most extreme eccentricity.'

'Surely eccentricity should not qualify someone for an insane asylum. There are many who would suggest that my dear husband is also eccentric. God forbid that I should lose him to such a fate.'

'Your humour is particularly sharp this morning. Did that soft bed give you a new lease on life?'

'Not the bed, Samuel. If my memory serves me, it was you who was asleep whilst I pined. Perhaps it is this fresh air?' Johanna inhaled deeply, savouring the scent of the forest on the spring air.

'Or perhaps it is time for another child to occupy your fertile mind.'

'You may be right. It would certainly be pleasant to have my husband spend time in our chambers when he has inclinations other than sleep.'

'Madam, please, the children should not hear such things.' Samuel's rebuke was hopelessly lost in his smile.

'If you hadn't noticed, the older children have deserted us for the delights of the forest. These two,' Johanna nodded at the toddler on Samuel's hip and the babe in her arms, 'are not paying any particular attention to us either. But if my husband wishes that I should be a little more circumspect in the middle of the forest, then so be it. Perhaps we should return to the subject of eccentricity?'

'Klockenbring's, I assume, as opposed to mine?'

'Oh most definitely, good sir, I already know all I need to about yours.'

Samuel looked across the meadow satisfied that he could still see all three of his older children as they ran along the edges of the forest. Above them the spire of the church in the village of Georgenthal rose beyond the trees.

'Klockenbring had most definitely been an eccentric man, but you will be pleased to know that it was not just because of this that he was committed. Apparently he went mad, and violently so, when he was dragged unwittingly into an immense scandal.' Samuel pondered this comment and then added, 'although he may not have been so unwitting.' Then he rushed on. 'Sadly the story is an indelicate one for the ears of a lady, and I'm not sure how to make the story acceptable.'

'I think you should try, Samuel,' Johanna replied quietly, her eyes narrowing.

Slowly a smile came to Samuel's face. 'Klockenbring was the victim of a scurrilous and almost obscene article written by the dramatist Kotzebue. The story was about an author, equally well-known, who Kotzebue accused of having been sent to prison for being the keeper of a brothel. Of course, none of this would have tipped Klockenbring over the edge, but then Kotzebue named Klockenbring as a close associate of the author. He went even further, and accused Klockenbring of having the most virulent venereal disease as a result of his association with the brothel owner. Kotzebue claimed the Minister of Police was not only involved in drunkenness and illicit sexual liaisons but was also guilty of fraud. The accusations were too much for Klockenbring.' Samuel paused to shake his head. 'That such an article could be published, and to have his high office and his beloved family at risk was what actually drove him mad.'

'But who would allow such an article to be printed if it is untrue? Why could Klockenbring not refute it through an article of his own?' Johanna asked, her eyes open wide at the story

'I agree. Why didn't he? Unless, of course, there was some truth in it.'

5

Samuel looked out of the open window of the coach. The hotel was almost in the centre of Gotha, in a side street just off the City Square. From his seat he could see the imposing structure of the Town Hall rising above his destination. He turned to the duke sitting opposite him. 'Your grace it has been a privilege to share this journey with you, I hope the remainder of yours is safe.'

'Thank you, but I think we should both be wishing the other good luck on the longer journey that we are just starting. You, sir, in particular.'

'I'm not sure it's luck I will be needing, but patience and lots of it. I must admit that I find the meeting in front of me a little daunting. I fear Frau Klockenbring may have to accept that her husband is not as innocent as she may think.'

'If that's all that's worrying you allow me to give you some advice. I have had the chance to meet with Frau Klockenbring on two occasions and I am still to truly understand what her motivations are. I have no doubt she wishes her husband to receive the best treatment, but I suspect that the underlying reason is to gratify the good lady's own ambitions.' the duke stopped abruptly. 'Perhaps I should leave it at that.'

Samuel shook the duke's hand with a new sense of disquiet.

'Thank you again, your grace, hopefully all will go well from this point.'

The duke's voice became more business like. 'I only have a short distance to travel. My driver will be out here waiting for you when you are ready to leave.'

Without another word Samuel climbed onto the single step the coachman had swung down. Carefully he stepped onto the road outside the hotel.

'Oh, I almost forgot,' the duke yelled out. 'The asylum has promised you any additional help you may need to manage your patient on the return journey.'

With a cry and a flick of the reins the coachman urged the four horses forward, the elegant carriage turning into the City Square and disappearing from Samuel's view. Reluctantly he turned to face the hotel entrance and took a deep breath.

A liveried servant opened the door.

'My name is Hahnemann, I am expected by Frau Klockenbring.'

'Please follow me, doctor.' The servant turned on his heel and led Samuel across the drawing room to a door on the far side. 'Madam is expecting you, but unfortunately she is suffering from a pounding headache and is still resting. She has asked that I present you in the bedroom, sir. Frau Klockenbring felt that would not cause you any concern given your training.'

The door stood ajar, the room darkened; Samuel assumed the drapes had been drawn to give some relief to the lady's condition. The servant tentatively knocked.

'It's open you fool, can't you see?' came the strident cry from within.

Stoically the servant avoided Samuel's eyes and pushed the door open. He announced Samuel in a soft whisper.

Again the voice cried out, insisting he speak up.

The servant raised an eyebrow at Samuel. 'Doctor Hahnemann is here to see you, Frau Klockenbring' his voice loud and clear.

Inside the room there was a rustle and then a pained voice called out softly. 'Please show my guest in, don't keep him waiting in the drawing room.'

Gingerly the servant pushed the door open, earning another cry from the bedroom. 'The light, oh please, quickly, Doctor Hahnemann, the pain is ... is... '

The servant offered Samuel a shrug of his shoulders and pulled the door closed.

Self-consciously Samuel cleared his throat. 'Frau Klockenbring, perhaps it would be better if I returned another time when you are not, er, indisposed.'

'Doctor, no, please, stay. It is so good of you to come. I have heard so much about you, and, oh what a relief. I mean, the treatment you outlined in your letter. How can I possibly start to thank you?'

Samuel could just make out the shape of the woman lying propped up on the large four poster bed, the bedclothes slightly crumpled.

'Such a blessed change from the agonies my poor, darling husband currently endures? He is such an intelligent man; sometimes his brilliance surprises me. Did I tell you in my letters that he is highly regarded as an author? So brilliant, but then so irritable. He so depends upon what others think of him.' A hint of anger entered the woman's voice. 'The doctor's say your fee is usurious, but I don't care. I wanted to meet you personally to say thank you.'

Samuel stood still, uncertain whether to interrupt or not.

'Oh dear, I must apologise for the poor manners of my welcome. I was struck down by this dreadful migraine when I tried to rise from my bed this morning. The hotel doctor has given me a pill that even my horses back home would have trouble swallowing, and do you think I can break the thing? Of course not, I doubt a hammer could perform that trick.' Frau Klockenbring's voice rose as she vented her displeasure on the hotel physician, then, just as quickly, became soft again. 'Please, doctor, come and sit by my side so I can at least see you whilst we talk. You should find a chair there.'

Cautiously Samuel crossed the darkened room in the direction of the bed. The loud crack could be heard clearly. With a gasp of pain Samuel clutched at his knee.

'Doctor, what have you done?' Frau Klockenbring's voice trembled with concern.

'It's all right, madam,' Samuel hissed through clenched teeth. 'I misjudged the distance and banged my knee on the end of the bed.' There was a rustle of bedclothes and a hand plucked at his sleeve, soft flesh pushing into his arm.

Sit down, doctor,' Frau Klockenbring held his arm firmly as she guided him to the chair. Samuel collapsed onto the seat, the woman's nightgown and a vast expanse of bosom looming above him in the gloom.

'Ma'am, perhaps I could suggest that you return to your bed,' he said nervously. 'In your condition you need to rest' Samuel had stopped rubbing his knee, grateful to see the woman was now back in her bed, the covers pulled up. Without warning, Frau Klockenbring leant towards Samuel, pushing a mountain of flesh only inches from his nose. He tore his eyes away from her heaving bosom. 'Madam, please! Please cover yourself or I will be forced to return to the drawing room whilst you dress appropriately.'

'Sir, I'm shocked. Surely my state of dress is of no concern to you? I would have thought your mind would be dealing with the symptoms of my wretched headache than with the size or shape of my bosom. I thought doctors were like men of the cloth, their minds filled with only pure thoughts. Oh this is too much, my poor head.' Frau Klockenbring collapsed backwards onto her pillow her hand flying to her mouth, tears springing to her eyes.

Samuel pulled a clean handkerchief from his sleeve and leant across the woman. 'Please, Frau Klockenbring, take this kerchief and wipe your eyes. It is bad enough that your husband should be indisposed without his good wife being so distressed. Please accept my apologies if I gave you cause for alarm.' Samuel said, searching his mind for what he had done to offend the lady so.

Frau Klockenbring reached out for the handkerchief. Her fingers touched Samuel's briefly as they folded around the cloth. Suddenly her hand reached out, dropping the handkerchief and closing around Samuel's. Before he could snatch it away she had clasped his palm to her bosom. Moaning and swooning she fell back on the bed, his hand clamped to her breast.

Samuel shot out his free hand to steady himself, horrified when he found both clasping at a mountain of flesh.

Through it all, Frau Klockenbring smiled blissfully.

'Madam ... Frau Klockenbring ... I must ... insist.' Each word struggled from Samuel's mouth as he tried to regain his balance.

A sudden shaft of light fell across the bed capturing Samuel's hands caressing Frau Klockenbring's breasts. He pulled with all his might just as the lady released her hold, her hands flying to her eyes to cover them. Samuel flew backward, missed the chair and sprawled across the carpet.

A hand reached out in the gloom pulling Samuel to his feet. Gratefully he allowed the servant to guide him to the doorway. As he neared safety, Frau Klockenbring called softly to him, her voice once more pleasant and cajoling.

'Thank you for coming, Doctor Hahnemann, I am sure you will take great care of my husband. Hopefully we can continue our discussions when I visit him.' The good lady then directed her tongue to the servant. 'See Doctor Hahnemann out, then return, your disobedience will have to be dealt with.'

Samuel turned to express his gratitude to the servant. The servant shook his head, his finger to his lips. Without a word he led Samuel to the front door of the suite.

'I wish you a safe journey, doctor.'

Again Samuel tried to speak, this attempt met with a shake of the young servant's head. 'Doctor, I can assure you,' the servant's whispered words were barely audible as he closed the door, 'some punishments are harsher than others.'

6

For the second time that morning Samuel stepped out from the carriage, his heart beating a fraction faster than it should have been. He looked up at the building, hating what he knew awaited him on the inside. His eyes took in the bars on the windows.

'I am not sure how long this will take,' Samuel called up to the coachman who had already regained his seat at the front of the carriage.

'No matter, doctor. I will take the horses across the way and find them some water.' The coachman touched his tricorn hat with the stock of his whip and urged the horses forward.

Samuel faced the stark brick building which housed the insane. He took a deep breath, wanting to settle the pace of his heart. Patting the front of his tunic to ensure the duke's letter of introduction was still secure, he mounted the stairs.

'Hey *scheisskopf*. You want to get in? Get to the end of the queue,' a man cried out.

Startled, Samuel looked up. He had paid no heed to the small queue of men and women impatiently shuffling along the wall. Each of them stared at Samuel. One of the women added her voice to the first man's cry, 'Yeah, *schweinhund*, too good to wait with folk like us, eh?'

The woman's dress was dirty and unkempt, her bosom jutted forward, exposing a smeared expanse of cleavage. Her hair was filthy, matted, her hand plucked nervously at the buttons on her bodice, the fingers soiled, the nails cracked.

'I assure you, ma'am, I was not trying to steal an advantage. I have business with the director of the asylum,' Samuel said, nerves adding a pretentious note to his voice.

'Asylum? This ain't no asylum, this 'ere's the local 'ouse of amusement,' the woman laughed, a slight note of hysteria creeping into her voice.

Samuel hesitated. His eyes darted to the front door and then across the road to where the duke's coachman had allowed the horses to rest. Then the purpose of the queue dawned on him. He clenched his fists.

'Out of my way,' Samuel shouted at the man in the front of the queue. 'You people disgust me. I'm not here to see some penny freak show.' Ignoring the cries from the first two men, Samuel shouldered his way to the door.

The first man clenched his fists and pushed his chest into Samuel, slowing his charge. The second man took courage from his friend and reached out to snatch at Samuel's sleeve.

With a crash, the front door to the building flew open. A huge man, his chest straining at the buttons of his woollen topcoat, stood on the step casting his glare across the rag taggle group of voyeurs. The two protagonists and the unkempt woman cringed away from the massive doorman.

'Doctor Hahnemann?' the man growled.

Samuel blinked and bent his head back to look up into the eyes of the man-mountain. He gulped, not trusting his voice, wondering if his constitution could take much more in one day.

The man-mountain gave a final glare at the queue. 'This way please. The director is waiting for you in his office.'

Self-consciously Samuel brushed at the sleeve that had so offended one of the men on the street. Squaring his shoulders, he stepped through the open door, his rescuer backing away to allow him through. The man slammed the door shut and pointed along a short corridor to where a metal grille barred further entry.

'This way, Herr doctor.' Without waiting, the man lumbered towards the grille. He lifted a key from his belt and slipped it into the keyhole in the square plate. It gave a solid clunk as it turned. He beckoned for Samuel to pass through, then locked the door behind him.

They were standing in a small vestibule, no more than twenty feet on all sides. The walls of the room were brick, the lintels above each door hewn blocks of stone. The room was cold and depressing and caused Samuel to shiver involuntarily. Three more doors opened off the anteroom. To his right stood a small desk with a single chair behind it.

'The director said you would have a letter from the duke?' The question was not impolite, but brusque.

Samuel reached into the inside pocket of his new jacket and retrieved the thick envelope. He handed it over without question.

The large man made no attempt to break the seal, satisfied that the wax carried the mark of the duke.

'You aren't the sensitive type, I hope. Some of the people in this place are like animals. You understand me, animals. Just stay with me, doctor. Ignore 'em if they try to approach you.'

Samuel nodded, knowing it would be pointless to admonish the man for his apparent prejudice.

The man lifted another key from the ring and opened the door opposite the entry, waving Samuel through as he did so. Samuel found himself in a courtyard, the blue sky at least welcoming.

Then he lowered his eyes.

Samuel's heart lurched at the scene before him. Several men and women sat around the perimeter of the courtyard, their backs against a wall that rose three stories. Barred windows overlooked the stone-flagged square at regular intervals.

Directly opposite Samuel, two men sat side by side staring at him. Beside them a woman slowly dropped her chin to her chest then, without pause, flung her head back, slamming it into the brick wall. The dull thud of bone striking the bricks echoed round the courtyard. Again she slammed her head against the bricks, and then again, each blow punctuated with a soft shake of her head. A tiny trickle of blood slid down the side of the woman's neck, her hair glistened red and patches of splattered blood painted the brickwork.

Samuel turned away in horror, trying to escape, but his eyes were trapped at the sight of another woman in the corner of the yard standing over a large iron grate. His heart leapt as she squealed with delight then flapped her skirt backwards and forwards across the iron bars below her. A tear appeared in Samuel's eye at the woman's mindless happiness. Suddenly a hand reached through the grille from below, grasping the woman's ankle. The woman shrieked with delight, allowing the hand to caress her ankle. Like a serpent the hand moved up the woman's leg until it could reach no further. The woman lifted the dress revealing her nakedness beneath. Squealing with delight she lowered herself onto the grate.

Ashamed, Samuel turned away, only to have his senses arrested by a sad tableau in another corner of the courtyard.

Three men sat at a table fashioned from a single block of stone. One was completely bald. The other two wore their hair long, tied at the back with dirty strips of cloth. With an exaggerated gesture the bald man slapped an imaginary card onto the top of the stone, his eyes glaring at the next man challenging him to follow suit. After a moment, the second man also slapped his hand on the rock before turning to the third man, a sneer on his face, daring the new player to do better. The third man glared balefully at his opponents then suddenly brushed the imaginary cards from the top of the slab. With a savage howl the bald man jumped up, smashed his head into the third man's face, sending him reeling backwards in pain. Blood poured from his forehead where the blow had split the skin.

'You see, doctor? The inmates are simply amusing themselves.' Samuel's guide nodded his head in the direction of the street. 'Those waiting outside pay a penny each to simply watch or to tease the animals in the zoo.'

The man-mountain didn't wait for a reply but moved off through the human debris towards a doorway on the opposite side of the courtyard. Samuel waited a moment, his stomach sick to the very core. A hand reached out and plucked at the hose on his leg. Instinctively he snatched his leg away, his heart beating rapidly as he looked down at the man who had reached out to him. He stumbled briefly then turned to follow his guide, catching up with him before he was halfway across the courtyard.

'Ah! You are still with me ...' The man reached out and opened the door without using a key. 'The director's office is just through here. I'm sure you'll find the surroundings a little more comfortable.'

'Welcome to our humble institution.' The director had introduced himself to Samuel as he'd taken the letter from the gatekeeper. 'Please have a seat, I will just make a notation of the duke's request so that we keep the records straight.' His words dripped with oil. 'Then I will take you to Herr Klockenbring.'

Samuel nodded, knowing that the director was probably as eager to be rid of him as Samuel was to leave.

'It is difficult for those who don't deal with the problem each day,' the director's tone was patronising, 'but let me assure you, my good doctor, that the animals locked up here are treated with the very best knowledge of the day. Even though there are some fools who think otherwise.'

'What do you mean by that, sir?' Samuel spluttered.

'Mean by what?' the director asked innocently.

'Your last remark.'

A veil slipped down over the director's eyes as the two men walked through a corridor bereft of any ornament or pictures. At regular intervals a stout door broke up the continuous length of bare-brick wall.

'Don't insult my intelligence, Doctor Hahnemann. I know your reputation. Like many charged with the burden of keeping these animals under control, I too have a medical background.

Your ideas, sir, are, I believe, preposterous. The doctrine you propose on bloodletting is anathema to me and to many of my colleagues.'

'How dare you ...'

Ignoring Samuel, the director continued. 'As for your far-fetched theories on dealing with the insane,' he shook his head angrily, 'that fool Becker is not capable of coming up with an original idea, never mind such ridiculous proposals as those. No, sir, I, and many of my colleagues, have seen your hand in that commentary and I say to you now, you will not succeed. You may have persuaded the duke to go along with your stupid experiment but I assure you that there are many waiting for it to fail so that we can be done with these stupid ideas with which you seem determined to ruin your career.'

Samuel held his tongue. He knew he would gain nothing by opposing the man's stupidity.

In stony silence the two men reached a cell at the end of the corridor. The director stepped forward and grasped the small knob on the metal slide, preparing to draw it back. 'Perhaps you would like to see what you are bringing upon yourself, Doctor Hahnemann, before I summon the men who will accompany you to the duke's lodge.' With the slide drawn open the director stood to one side to allow Samuel his first view of his patient.

Herr Klockenberg, the respected Minister of Police and Secretary to the Chancellor of Hanover, sat on a rough stone bench against the far wall.

Above his head a window framed the beautiful spring day. Bars sliced the sky into long parallels, their length buried deep in the stone. Light poured into the room in stark contrast to the darkness Samuel had expected. Samuel bit down harshly on his lip to prevent the cry of surprise and revulsion that threatened to escape from his throat.

The esteemed Minister of Police was as naked as the day he was born. His face and skin were covered in large, scaly spots. The hair on his head hung in filthy clumps while the hair on his chest and at his groin was equally as filthy and crawling with lice. Chains stretched from the man's wrists to rings affixed into the brick wall on either side of the stone bench.

The light hid nothing. Samuel could see blotches of red at each wrist where the manacles had bitten into the skin. The man's feet were also manacled to a ring attached to the bench. A short length of chain allowed him to move no more than a few feet from his current position.

Samuel turned to the director. 'How do you explain this, sir? This man has not been treated with even the scantest respect.'

'Respect? What kind of demented fool are you, Hahnemann?' the director's voice lashed back. 'We can do nothing about this man's condition because he will not allow us. At best we can cleanse him by throwing a pail of water over him. When he is subdued, which I assure you is infrequent, his minders dress him, but he refuses to remain in that state; tearing the clothes from his own back as if they bedevil him. The chains are there for his own protection as much as ours, and you would be well counselled not to try your futile heroics or so-called gentle methods. Bah, gentle methods indeed! You can see that this man is a danger to himself and to others and he must be treated accordingly.'

'I see no such thing. I see a man who is responding to this cruelty in the only way one can expect him to. You treat him like a wild animal and expect culture in return?' Samuel's eyes narrowed. 'Has this man been subjected to the horizontal board?' Samuel knew the answer as soon as the director dropped his eyes. 'So how many times has he been subjected to that abomination?' Samuel pressed. 'What else? Emetics? Tell me, what diabolical measures of nauseating medicines have been forced down his throat?' Samuel paused to catch his breath. 'Open this door ... please.'

Grudgingly, the director took a large key from his pocket and unlocked the heavy door.

A vile stench caused Samuel to gag. He pulled his handkerchief from his sleeve to cover his nose. The sight of it made him blush at the memory of the wretched man's semi-naked wife. Placing the kerchief to his face, Samuel advanced into the room. 'He must be washed before his journey. We cannot expect to travel such a distance with this ... this stench.'

'So you are human after all, doctor, you suffer the same frailties we poor mortals do. There is still hope for us then.'

'You waste your sarcasm, sir. Yes, I am human. I smell, I see and I shit like other men. There is no shame in that, sir, but there is shame in treating men thus. I would never allow an insane man to be punished by blows, or any other kind of corporal chastisement. There is no understanding of the punishment where there is no responsibility. I suspect these people are only rendered the worse by such rough and callous treatment. Please call your men and tell them to bring some warmed water. I will wash the man myself if no-one else has the nerve to.'

7

The man-mountain had a name.
The director had made no effort to introduce Samuel to the two men detailed to travel with him to Georgenthal. Samuel had overhead the director's whispered instructions, catching the name Heinz twice as the director poked the big man in the chest and impressed on him the necessity that he return with all haste.

A canvas smock wrapped the Minister for Police in a cocoon, his arms trapped against his body. Heinz sat next to the patient with Samuel opposite. His fellow gaoler sat next to Samuel.

With a deep sigh Samuel called out to the coachman that all was well and that they should leave immediately for the peace and beauty of Georgenthal.

The four men sat in silence as they rocked and bumped along the road. Samuel was forced to clutch for a handhold at the worst of the road conditions. He watched with admiration as Heinz ensured his charge did not roll about, and wondered if the man would have the strength to continue for the three hours of their nine-mile journey.

After an hour, the road started to rise through the gentle foothills of the Thuringer Wald; the landscape switching between glades of forest and long expanses of meadow that dipped and swayed under the weight of the spring flowers.

Samuel glanced across at Klockinbring, who appeared to be sleeping.

He was surprised to see Heinz appraising him through half closed eyes. Samuel felt no fear of the man simply because of his size, but he felt strangely intimidated by this scrutiny.

'Is there something wrong? Have I a fly on my face, or perhaps something more disquieting?' Samuel asked.

A soft smile appeared on the man mountain's lips, followed by a slow shake of his head. The second gaoler's eyes were closed.

Without warning, Herr Klockenbring swivelled his head away from the window and with a savage grunt buried his teeth in the shoulder of the man beside him. Instantly awake, the gaoler next to Samuel launched himself across the short space, his fist catching Klockenbring in the side of the head. Ignoring the blow, the Minister for Police maintained his grip. The gaoler drew back his fist ready to deliver a second blow.

'Stop!' The cry came from the Heinz, catching Samuel off guard as he also readied to shout. 'Hitting him will not shake him; he just buries his teeth deeper.' Heinz said through gritted teeth. He reached over with his free hand and placed a huge thumb on Klockenbring's neck just beside the man's ear. Slowly he began to apply pressure. Samuel could see the strain on the man's digit as it held its place. Klockenbring's jaw relaxed, the man's eyes went blank and then closed in a dead faint. Carefully Heinz took his thumb away from the pressure point and lifted the hand to gently push his assailant's forehead away until it rested peacefully on the side of the carriage.

'Are you all right? Let me see how bad the damage is.' Samuel spoke quietly but deliberately, impressed with the way the man had managed the attack, yet concerned, his private fears unspoken.

'I don't think he broke the skin, Doctor Hahnemann,' the big man responded. My leather vest may look like someone has mistaken it for a new season's apple, but I think it has saved me from the worst.'

'Nevertheless, better safe than sorry, Heinz ... do you mind if I call you Heinz?'

The man-mountain shook his head. 'I will ask the coachman to stop, it may make the inspection a little more comfortable.'

Samuel insisted that the coachman collect some water from a nearby stream so that he could carefully wash the injured shoulder. Thanks to the leather jerkin the skin had only been grazed but Samuel wanted to take every precaution. If he was right, and he suspected he was from the signs he had seen on the man's skin, Klockenbring was riddled with syphilis.

For the moment he had no intention of alarming Heinz, but he knew he would be much happier if he could observe him for a few days to settle his doubts. The second guard had wanted to fix a gag to their patient to ensure there would be no repeat. Samuel refused, and was again surprised when the man-mountain concurred.

'I suspect your shoulder will be black and blue by the morning, but I would be pleased if you would again allow me to cleanse and bathe the area before you return to Gotha. Herr Klockenbring could be diseased and I think it prudent that we take every precaution.'

'Diseased?' Heinz's eyes showed no alarm.

'I am not sure, but I suspect that part of his madness is due to a sickness of the body. I don't wish to alarm you, so I should be cautious in what I say.'

Heinz nodded. He too had suspected the man was carrying some disease. 'If he does have a venereal disease of some type, doctor, what is the likelihood that he has passed it to me?'

'I think slight, very slight, but I must admit that our knowledge is still not as it should be. So called *learned* books on pathology claim that disease is propagated by the application of the infected material to the skin or to a wound. But it is not proven. Does the venereal disease pass through the saliva of one to the blood of another by a bite such as the one you have received? Perhaps. The most careful and prompt washing of the genitals does not protect the philanderer from syphilis if that disease is present in the host, or should I say hostess,' Samuel added with a self-conscious smile.'

'And if this disease — lets call it syphilis so we can consider the worst of the options you have entertained, Doctor Hahnemann — if I were to contract such a disease from this man's attack. Can you cure it?'

'Most assuredly, Heinz. As I believe I can cure Herr Klockenbring of his so-called insanity by treating his physical condition.'

Both of Klockenbring's gaolers looked at Hahnemann in surprise.

'This man,' the gaoler said pointing at Klockenbring, 'he is insane, mad. That is why he was in the asylum. This is fool's talk. He does not suffer from some malaise which has made him mad. He *is* mad.' The gaoler turned his head away from Samuel in disgust and stared out of the coach window.

Samuel studied the back of the man's head for a moment before replying. 'When we reach the duke's hunting lodge I will enlist your aid one more time to remove Herr Klockenbring's restraints. It is my intention to observe and treat the man, not to punish him. If, sir,' Samuel looked pointedly at the back of the head of the second gaoler, 'if in your mind that makes me equally insane then I shall have to live with your condemnation and, I suspect, your ridicule.'

8

'Doctor Hahnemann, a word please.' Heinz gently rested his hand on Samuel's arm.

The two men were alone in the corridor outside Klockenbring's room. The man-mountain's truculent confederate had gone in search of the kitchen, his temper slightly mollified by Samuel's offer of sustenance. A few minutes before, the two gaolers had removed the patient's restraining jacket, leaving him sitting quietly in his new quarters.

'How is your shoulder?' Samuel asked.

'Sore. And I think you are right, it will be the colour of midnight by tomorrow.' Heinz had allowed Samuel to again wash the affected area, although the graze had already faded and little blood was in evidence around the broken skin.

'You should take great care of your leather jerkin,' Samuel said with a smile. 'Treasure it as you would a precious child; it may prove to be your talisman for a long life.'

'Doctor, I wonder if I may speak bluntly?'

Samuel looked up at the huge man towering over him. 'Of course. Come to my quarters, we can have more privacy there?'

'Here is fine, doctor. My words will only take a few moments and my friend's stomach will keep him occupied for a while.' Heinz paused, collecting his thoughts. 'Doctor, my work at the asylum earns me my keep, but I silently weep when I see the ravages inflicted on the inmates. I bite my tongue because it is not easy to come by work. Yet I hope that in some small way I ease the suffering of some of the people there. I have also taught myself how to deal peacefully with their violent outbursts.'

'Yes, I was very impressed on the coach. It was much more appropriate than the action proposed by your colleague.'

'Unfortunately it is not always possible to ease the suffering of the poor wretches forced to live there.' Heinz shrugged. 'But a job is a job.'

'So, what is it that I can help with?'

'I wondered if you could use someone who has some knowledge and some skills in dealing with these poor folk. I understand that the duke's benevolence is to extend beyond the treatment of Herr Klockenbring.' Heinz rushed on, 'The article that appeared in *Der Anzeiger* suggested a nursing home for mental patients of the better classes. That suggests more than one patient is expected.' Heinz paused before finishing lamely, 'I could be of some value to you, sir.'

Samuel regarded the man carefully. He was much more articulate than the first impression he'd gained at the asylum, and he was impressed with his gentle manner and his way of dealing with circumstances.

'Regrettably, I cannot confirm what the future holds for our small nursing home. For the moment we have one patient. We have had no other approaches. Perhaps even the better classes prefer to turn their backs on insanity, or they are not prepared to pay the necessary fees.' Samuel shook his head sadly, 'Even if I could offer you a job, how long would it last? I am confident that we will cure Herr Klockenbring. When he goes home to his wife, what then of a nursing home without patients?'

'I would gladly take the risk of short-term tenure to watch you work your magic. I can earn my keep, I promise. I have turned my hand to many parts in my life and I do not bring the added burden of a family that requires feeding and schooling.'

Samuel rubbed his chin. 'Heinz, I cannot in all honesty

promise you something that is not in my power to give. But I will promise you this.' A spark came to the eyes of the man-mountain as he listened. 'At this point in time, my wife and I are the only people employed to care for Herr Klockenbring. We are charged with caring for ourselves, and that means my wife will take responsibility for our cooking and cleaning, including Herr Klockenbring's quarters. Should circumstances change, or should I discern that the patient is too violent for my own safety, I will persuade the duke to offer you a contract. But I'm afraid that is the best I can offer at this moment. I wish it were more.'

Samuel and Johanna stood in the forecourt of the hunting lodge and watched the coachman turn his four steeds back in the direction of the city.

Samuel had tried to persuade Heinz and his partner to stay the night, but the second gaoler had reminded Heinz of their promise to the Director. With a quiet word to the coachman to be careful and to either stay at the duke's castle in Gotha or find other lodgings, Samuel waved the group away.

He took his wife's hand and turned towards the house, anxious to begin to prove his detractors wrong.

A loud crash made them look up. Klockenbring stood framed against the first floor window, blood dripping from his arm. Jagged shards of glass threatened more damage as the man waved a belligerent fist at the departing coach.

Samuel broke into a run, his legs carrying him across the steps three at a time. His heart pumped furiously as he wondered if he might yet regret his refusal of help.

9

Samuel peered through the small spy-hole before unlocking the door. The Minister for Police sat on a stool in front of a majestic grand piano, its size and grandeur dominating the pleasantly furnished room. Bars on the two windows were the only evidence of incarceration.

Klockenbring was naked. His clothes were scattered across a nearby couch. Blood dripped from his arm, yet he seemed unaware of it and did nothing to staunch the flow. Through the spy-hole, Samuel could see Klockenbring's lips moving, but no sound reached him through the thick door. Steeling himself, Samuel turned the key and gently pushed the door open. His heart hammered in his chest. Klockenbring turned, a gentle satisfied smile interrupting his recitation. Suddenly he jumped to his feet, his bloodied arm waving in Samuel's direction, droplets of blood splattering across the arm of the couch.

Alarmed, Samuel waited in the doorway. The two men stared at each other for a long time. Finally, the Minister for Police resumed his recitation, his legs and arms spread wide, his voice taking on a magnificent timbre.

> '*O Muses, O high genius, now assist me!*
> *O memory, that didst write down what I saw,*

> *Here thy nobility shall be manifest!*
> *And I began: 'Poet, who guidest me,*
> *Regard my manhood, if it be sufficient,*
> *Ere to the arduous pass thou dost confide me.'*

Unbidden, Samuel dropped his eyes at the poet's instructions before wrenching them away in embarrassment.

> *Thou sayest, that of Silvius the parent,*
> *While yet corruptible, unto the world*
> *Immortal went, and was there bodily.*

Amazed at the performance, Samuel moved closer. Dante himself would have been proud of the delivery and the word-perfect recall. Klockenbring continued his recitation unaware of the blood that dripped from his arm onto his thighs. A streak of vermilion blossomed between large scabs on his chest as he swung his arm in a sweeping gesture more suited to the theatrics of the stage.

> *'To men of intellect unmeet it seems not;*
> *For he was of great Rome, and of her empire*
> *In the empyreal heaven as father chosen;'*

Samuel's knowledge of the *Inferno*'s sweeping damnation was enough to admire the quality of Klockenbring's performance. Yet, admirable as it may be, Samuel worried that the man would soon collapse from loss of blood unless he could tend the wound.

> *The which and what, wishing to speak the truth,*
> *Were stablished as the holy place, wherein*
> *Sits the successor of the greatest Peter.'*

As calmly as he could, Samuel placed his hand on Klockenbring's shoulder, holding his breath as he pushed gently. Klockenbring allowed Samuel to ease him down onto the couch. But as his naked buttocks touched the brocade he jumped up, his arm sweeping out, his voice rising with the telling.

> *'Upon this journey, whence thou givest him vaunt,*
> *Things did he hear, which the occasion were*
> *Both of his victory and the papal mantle.'*

The recitation halted mid-verse. Without warning, Klockenbring lunged across the floor and grasped a writing slate lying on the rug. He swiped his hand beneath the couch and pulled out a stick of chalk. Ignoring the drops of blood scattered across the polished boards, he sat down on the floor and began chalking rapidly across the surface of the writing slate.

Samuel rose to his feet unable to make out what Klockenbring was scribbling. He cast his eyes around the room, seeking something with which to wrap Klockenbring's wounds. His eyes came to rest on a cloth beside the bowl of water left for their patient's ablutions. Samuel snatched up the cloth. With a single bite, he broke the stitched hem and tore it into strips.

He returned to the couch where he caught a glimpse of Klockenbring's writings. The slate was covered in algebraic formulae that began with a simple theorem but then exploded into complex and detailed solutions.

Samuel read the first two. They seemed familiar.

$$a = bq_1 + r_1, \text{ with } 0 \; r_1 < b$$
$$b = r_1 q_2 + r_2, \text{ with } 0 \; r_2 < r_1$$

Klockenbring was deep in thought, musing over the scientific masterpiece on his knee, the deep cut in his forearm ignored. On closer inspection Samuel breathed a small sigh, judging the cut less life threatening than he had initially thought. He was relieved to see the blood already starting to congeal at the edges.

'I need to stitch your cut, Herr Klockenbring,' Samuel said, 'else it will continue to bleed and I fear you will weaken before you can finish your masterpiece of science.'

Klockenbring lifted his eyes from the slate and looked at the wound. 'Do what you must, but hurry, I need to finish,' he snapped.

Without hindrance, Samuel wrapped the arm with the strip of cloth, hoping the Minister for Police would remain quiet for the few minutes it would take him to get needle and gut from his medical case.

'I don't think I have ever heard a more correct recitation. And in English, for goodness sake. No-one informed me that the man was a linguist.' Samuel's voice betrayed his amazement. 'Even the misguided fools who studied Literature at the university could not have effected a better performance.' He watched his wife thread silk onto a needle, the image prompting his memory of the needle and gut as it had pierced Klockenbring's arm. Samuel smiled grimly to himself. When he had returned, the slate had been cleaned of its algebra, replaced by a language that Samuel recognised but could not read, Hebrew being of little import in his work as a translator.

'Will he suffer from it?' Johanna asked without looking up from the detail of her embroidery.

'He will carry the scar, but I think that is of little consequence given his condition.' Samuel smiled at his own humour, albeit fleetingly. 'I must admit that I am still somewhat shaken by the experience. It was only with the grace of God that the man remained relatively calm. Perhaps I should be grateful for his amazing performance for it kept his mind off other things.'

'You fear his violence?' Johanna looked up, concern in her eyes.

'Most assuredly. He is a bigger man than I. That would not normally cause me concern, but his wretched condition means that the unexpected has become the expected. Frau Klockenbring indicated that her husband was a very learned man, but also a boastful one. Apparently he claimed intimate acquaintance with many dignified personages, although there is no proof to verify his claims. I believe the man's performance today is symptomatic of that same ego.'

'Perhaps you were hasty in despatching the man who offered you his assistance?' Johanna replied, lifting her head.

Samuel nodded, grateful for his wife's concern. 'I am convinced, my sweet Elise, that the only way to treat this man is through the development of a rapport between physician and patient. I was alarmed at the injury Herr Klockenbring did to himself this afternoon, but a glimmer of the man's true self was revealed. He allowed me to repair his wound with a measure of contrition that suggested he knew he was responsible for his own pain.'

Samuel stopped to ponder his next words, a hand absently rubbing his chin. 'Pain and punishment inflicted by others must be avoided at all costs. What I observed Heinz do today was most assuredly a more gentle manner than his colleague was prepared to display, but I could not predict how Herr Klockenbring would react in the presence of such an intimidating man whose sheer size would frighten the sane.'

'But what of your own protection?' his wife implored.

'This man is ill. He does not know what he is doing, so he should not receive punishment for doing it. I must win the man's trust and confidence to be able to treat him as I intend. To do that I must show him that I am unconcerned, that I see him as a reasonable human being.'

'I think I would like my husband to return to our quarters each evening in one piece, even if it is only to help with the chores.' Johanna allowed a small smile to appear on her lips.

Samuel smiled back at his wife. 'Rest assured; I will not risk your tongue for the sake of the patient's treatment. If I truly believe that Klockenbring is a danger to my well-being, I will have the coachman travel to Gotha at the earliest opportunity with a letter of offer.'

10

Samuel stood at the kitchen table. His hands and arms were covered in flour. A smudge of white showed on his cheek where his hand had reached to still an itch. Johanna stood next to him rolling pastry, two pie dishes at her elbow. Beside her, Henrietta nursed the sleeping Caroline, the remnants of a bowl of stewed apple on the end of the table. The rest of the children had already been fed and put to bed.

'You are very quiet this evening. Are you angry that I would ask for your help? I know you must be tired after managing your patient this past week.'

Samuel shook his head gently. 'I'm sorry if I appear distracted. For someone who sits and does nothing very much all day, I am surprisingly tired.'

'I must admit to some intrigue as to what you actually are doing, but, I suspect, that it is not "nothing very much".'

'Well, that's the truth of it,' Samuel replied. 'I spend my days sitting in the corner of his room, watching him. Then in the evening I spend time writing up my notes or, when you ask for it, helping you with the household duties.' Samuel held his white-coated hands up, a wry smile on his face. 'I can only apologise that our patient has added to them so. I cannot fathom how any man could consume ten pounds of bread in a single sitting, or consume two of your pies, when one would feed most for a week.' Samuel reflected on the dough he was kneading. 'Tomorrow I will have to send the coachman to Gotha for more supplies again.'

'Stop worrying about me. I can cope with the cooking. You are the one I worry about; each day I await your return, fearful that it may be with a broken limb or a nasty cut where your patient has chosen to lash out.'

'He is certainly violent. He has destroyed several pieces of furniture. Three times this week I have arrived to find him naked, his clothes ripped and strewn across the floor. This morning his bowl was smashed against the hearth. Yet when I approached him the man was in tears, staring forlornly at his wrists. I feared that he had injured himself, but the marks he showed me were old.' Samuel paused and stared at the dough. 'They were the scars inflicted by his gaolers in the asylum. Oh, if only you could have seen the look of fear and pain in his eyes, Elise, you would understand why I no longer worry that the man will injure himself.'

Johanna watched her husband pound the dough with the heels of his hands. She kept her own counsel, waiting for her husband to continue.

'I am more certain than ever that people who suffer in this way must be given reason for hope.' Samuel said. 'Physicians caring for the insane must have sympathy for their patients' unreasonable outbreaks of anger and their pitiful state, because it is only through sympathy that I feel we can begin our journey of cure.'

Johanna glanced anxiously at Samuel's frenzied hands.

Samuel continued, his voice getting louder. 'I am further convinced that it is absurd to view disease as separate from the living whole, as so many of our doctors do. Disease is not a hidden evil lurking in the body to be expunged by foul methods of evacuation or blood-letting. Or in the case of the so called insane, to be purged through whippings or banishment to dark and foul dungeons.'

Samuel picked up the rolled lump of dough and thumped it back onto the table.

'It is beholden on physicians to understand the symptoms of their patient's malaise. Not just make some imperious diagnosis that fits their so called cure, or to give them an excuse to administer huge quantities of medications that can only benefit the pockets of the doctors or the apothecaries.'

Samuel lifted the dough and shaped to pound it back to the board but stopped as he recognised the soft touch of his wife's hand on his cheek. Slowly he lifted his eyes to Johanna's face and her soft smile. She appraised his shirt. Self-consciously Samuel followed her gaze. Flour dust covered his shirt and pants. At his feet the floor was covered in white. He smiled sheepishly and dropped the dough limply back onto the table. He lifted his hands to wipe them on his shirt, the look of menace on Johanna's face causing him to stop half way. Finally Johanna could hold back no longer, her face dissolving into smiles. Then a laugh broke from her lips.

'My dearest husband,' she stuttered between laughs, 'I suspect that your anger guarantees we will have the lightest, sweetest bread in all of Georgenthal to tempt your patient with in the morning.'

Johanna had retired after settling the baby. Samuel sat at his desk. The notes he had made the previous day took his attention.

> The patient once again displayed a ferocious power of mind. At one moment he spoke as a judge passing sentence. The next he was Hector quoting chapter and verse from the Iliad. This performance lasted, at the very least, twenty minutes and, although I don't profess to know the poem intimately, it seemed to be the most magnificent, albeit incomplete, recitation of the role. Even then he was still not done, returning to his previous

dissertation in Hebrew. This time I recognised part of the incantation heard at my only visit to the synagogue in Leipzig.

Without warning, a crash sounded from above. Samuel jumped, his head jerking towards the door of the small room he had taken as his study. Again he heard the noise, combined with the tinkle of piano. He ran to the door, grimacing at another crash. In only a few strides he was on the stairs heading for Klockenbring's quarters.

He turned the key in the lock and flung the door open. Klockenbring stood naked in the centre of the room. In his hand he held one of the legs of the grand piano, the rest of the instrument lay in dismembered bits on the floor around him. Klockenbring's glare became darker as he regarded Samuel.

'Ah, my eminent observer. Were you the one responsible for the sourness of this obscenity?' Klockenbring indicated the destruction at his feet. 'I only played a single note and the noise was like a cacophony of the worst kind, a screeching worse than anything that the abomination in Gotha could muster. Was that your doing, sir?'

Samuel looked from the man's face to the jumbled mess of timber, ivory and wire. 'I have to admit Herr Klockenbring that I am not particularly musical and I have little understanding of the mechanics of such a complex instrument, certainly not enough to change the piano from its normal tone.'

'But you misunderstand me, sir,' Klockenbring said indignantly. 'It is the abomination's so-called correct tone that is so offensive.' Abruptly Klockenbring pitched the piano leg he was holding into the middle of the pile of debris. Samuel picked it up, surprised at the weight of it.

'Leave it.'

'I think it would be preferable if I cleared the pieces away.'

'I said leave it. I will repair it. I did the damage. Please, leave me now, I wish to sleep.'

11

'Your grace, I would ask that you not insist on meeting with Herr Klockenbring. He has made good progress but I fear that a distraction at this stage may undo the good work. I have already been forced to write to his wife urging her to stay away.'

'The good lady wished to visit and you declined her?' Surprise showed on the face of the Duke of Gotha.

Samuel nodded. 'For the good of the patient, your grace. Frau Klockenbring wrote of her intention to spend the winter with her husband. I had to be at my most persuasive because I truly believe it is only through complete solitude that I have been able to lead the patient's mind onto the right path.'

'You are saying, sir, that the man is cured?' The duke's eyebrows lifted in astonishment.

'Not fully, but we have travelled a long way down the path. The eruptions of his skin have cleared and the excessive demands he made in the first few months have declined.' A smile came to Samuel's lips. 'He now only eats four or five pounds of bread a day, and one pie.'

'I'm sorry, Doctor Hahnemann, but I fail to see ...'

'In the early days of his cure he suffered from the most extreme gluttony. In fact I was forced at one stage to administer twenty-five grains of tartar emetic to ease his discomfort.' The admission caused Samuel to wince.

'I am impressed, sir. He has been in your care no more than six months.'

'Seven months almost to the day.'

The duke acknowledged the correction, an expression of amazement fixed to his face. 'Then seven months. How much longer do you think you will need to treat him?'

'The signs are very positive. I suspect we will probably be able to make a more complete announcement within the next month or two.'

'If it is not possible to meet with the gentleman, is it possible to see the amazing evidence of your cure?'

'I am still reluctant to announce that success, your grace. But, yes, there is a small spy-hole in the door. I will show you.'

Together they climbed the stairs to the first floor where Samuel waved the duke to the door of the room. The spy-hole was set two thirds of the way up in the solid timber. With a glance at Samuel, the duke bent to bring his eye to the viewing device.

'What in hell's name? What is that monstrous contraption he is sitting at?'

Samuel smiled as he waited for the duke to drag his eyes from the spy-hole. 'Well, what is it, man?'

'I think it is his piano, your grace.'

'Piano? Don't be absurd. Take a look yourself. How can that thing be called a piano?'

Samuel placed his eye to the thin tube and looked into the room. Herr Klockenbring sat at the strange contraption that Samuel had become acquainted with over the past few months. A smile slowly crept onto his face. The Minister for Police had been as good as his word, or almost. What had risen from the pile of debris and destruction had not quite assumed the beauty of a phoenix, nor did it emit the same sweet tones of the deceased instrument, but Samuel had to admit that Klockenbring had used all the parts, albeit to his own design and intent. No two parts of the original had been rejoined as their original maker had designed. Perhaps the keyboard managed something of its original relationship with the player, who was now seated on the edge of the couch, his right hand raised to play a note. Samuel could not see Klockenbring's base hand, the angle of the keyboard obliterating it from view. Samuel turned away from the spy-hole.

'Yes, I was right, your grace, that is his piano.' Before the duke could bluster further, Samuel held up a hand. 'Your grace, please let me explain.'

The servant left the drawing room. Beside the duke's elbow sat a decanter of whisky. Samuel joined him with a glass of wine.

'So you expect me to believe that Herr Klockenbring sits and plays that ... that thing. How could anyone call it a piano? Or perhaps you have caught a little of the man's disease.'

'Oh I can assure you, your grace, that is most unlikely.' Samuel smiled and then waved his hand in a dismissive manner. 'Herr Klockenbring explained it to me not long after he had rebuilt it in his style. He told me that he had been forced to do so to find a complementary note.'

'A complementary note? Please don't mock me.'

'Your grace, that is the last thing I would do. They were his words. He has even given it a name. He calls it his proslambanomenon.'

'His what? Clearly the man is still mad.'

Samuel's smile widened. The duke finally saw the absurdity of his remark and broke into a smile.

'Well, doctor, my congratulations. Here's to your health and that of your patient.' Samuel lifted the glass to his mouth and drank. 'Unfortunately I am also the bearer of some disturbing news that your friend Herr Becker shared with me a few days ago.'

'Disturbing news, your grace? What could be disturbing at this time?' asked Samuel.

'It appears that the medical profession are once again up in arms about your good self.'

'About me? I have been very circumspect over the past few months. I've even refrained from sending letters or articles to publishers.'

'It appears that they have taken great offence at the fee you have sought from Frau Klockenbring.'

'My fee? What business is that of the doctors of Gotha?'

'Absolutely none, but that doesn't prevent them poking their noses where they don't belong. In fact their attack is particularly bitter and scathing of what they call a usurious fee. Much is being made of their attack, particularly in letters to editors.'

'This is completely unjust. I asked for and was granted a fee of one thousand thalers from Frau Klockenbring. She was most comfortable with it. She and her husband are in a good financial position; they can afford it.'

'It is not my place to query your remuneration, I am simply bringing the matter to your attention.'

Samuel rose to his feet and paced the floor, wringing his hands in front of him. 'For more than six months I have devoted myself to the cure of this man. My wife, my family, has also been required to share the burden of my preoccupation. And now we are so close to a cure. Not one of those physicians could cure him, and that included Wichmann, for whom I otherwise have the greatest respect.' Samuel's voice rose as he considered the injustice of his fellow doctors.

'Please calm yourself, Samuel. You have a good friend in Herr Becker. He has already taken up your defence, not through the press but in the Freemason halls where he carries a great deal of influence, perhaps even more than my own. Your credentials will be even stronger when you are able to announce the recovery of Klockenbring.'

Samuel sank back into his chair. 'Your grace, I am most appreciative of you bringing this warning to me, but I fear that I have made some life-long enemies who will find every reason to criticise. I don't think that will change whether I cure the Minister for Police or not.'

PART TWO

SAXONY 1793 – 1794

12

The huge man climbed down from his seat and looped the reins over a small metal hook.

'My friend, I had no idea.' Samuel's face broke into a broad grin as soon as he recognised Heinz. 'When Herr Becker agreed to arrange our transport it never occurred to me that you would be our driver. I must admit with some guilt that I assumed you still worked at the asylum.'

Samuel's outstretched hand disappeared inside the expanse of Heinz's palm. 'You have no reason to feel guilty, Doctor Hahnemann, I understood very well the position you were in, and it seems that your anxiety was well founded.'

'Yes, I am afraid so. I was always concerned that we would not find others prepared or able to afford the support and treatment we provided.'

Heinz extended his hand to Johanna then turned back to face Samuel. 'Your cure of Klockenbring is on everyone's lips in Gotha. Although there are some who would have people believe that it was a miracle or holy intervention that enabled him to return to his wife and his home.'

Johanna saw the blood infuse her husband's face and placed a gentle hand on his arm. Without looking at her, Samuel nodded, forcing a smile to his lips.

'But what of you? What prompted you to leave the asylum and take up this work?'

'Well, in some ways I owe that to you, sir.'

'To me? I don't understand. I turned you down when you were in need.' A frown creased Samuel's brow.

'What you were doing got me thinking.' Heinz smiled at the perplexed look of his host. 'All the way back to Gotha I could not get your ideas for treating the insane from my head. They made me even more disenchanted with the ways of the asylum and the sadistic ways of the people running it. So I made the decision to seek employment elsewhere. Not long after, I was fortunate to meet Councillor Becker. Presumptuously I inquired if there was any word on your progress. Naturally he asked me of my interest, and I have to admit I unburdened myself on the poor Councillor. As fortune had it, he knew of a man who was looking for a driver and a labourer in his fledgling freight business. I applied the next day, and to my surprise was offered the job immediately.'

Samuel reached out and grasped the big man's arm with delight. 'Congratulations, my friend,' he smiled, 'but I don't think I can take any of the credit for that set of circumstances.'

'Ah, but there is more.' The big man's eyes sparkled and then softened. 'The owner of the business was killed in an accident on the road to Hanover a week after I joined. With only a young boy and no family to help her, his widow accepted Herr Becker's assistance to help sell the business. So without money or a job I was once again faced with an uncertain future. Until completely out of the blue Herr Becker offered to finance my taking over the business.'

'Then I am even more delighted for you, even though I share the sadness of the poor widow.'

Heinz nodded his agreement. 'Fortunately her bereavement was relatively short, for she has since consented to become my wife.' The twinkle returned to his eyes. 'So I am blessed with both her nurturing care and her knowledge and experience in the business.'

'They say good luck comes in threes.'

'There was more to it than luck. Herr Becker told me that you had written to him extolling my virtues, advising him that I was seeking employment.' Heinz left the sentence unfinished, raising an eyebrow in Samuel's direction. 'I doubt that Herr Becker would have listened to the doorman of an insane asylum unless something had prompted him. Nor would he have subsequently offered that same man financial assistance unless he had good reason to trust my references.'

Samuel waved his hand, dismissing the thanks with barely concealed embarrassment. 'Don't be absurd, Heinz. Herr Becker is a man of his own consideration. My letter was simply a courtesy to our conversation. I have no doubt that what you have achieved is because of your own commitment. Please, enough of this talk, I refuse to acknowledge that I did anymore than pass on the measure of our conversation.'

Heinz smiled at Johanna. His smile became broader as his gaze embraced the pile of belongings stacked in front of the duke's hunting lodge.

'Then, let's get to business.' Heinz winked at Johanna. 'I have heard rumours that the fee you charged Herr Klockenbring and his good wife would buy my business five times over, so I have no hesitation in asking a fair and equitable price for the journey we are about to undertake. I think thirty thalers would be fair.'

Samuel turned from inspecting his belongings, a shocked expression on his face. 'Thirty thalers to carry us from here to Molschleben. That is ...' He looked from Heinz to his wife. Both of them were grinning broadly.

'What?' Samuel asked in exasperation. As realisation dawned on him, Samuel became sheepish, recognising his earlier lack of grace. 'I truly do believe, sir, that your own honesty and integrity would have won over even the hard-headed Becker. But, yes, he is a friend, and a good one, and I am pleased that he took some cognisance of my observations.' Samuel rubbed his hands together. 'Now, some serious discussion on the matter of a fair price.'

At last the family were settled into the lead coach. Samuel and young Friedrich sat up beside Heinz while Johanna and the remaining four children were ensconced inside.

With the giant's help it had taken little more than an hour to load their belongings onto the two coaches. Most of it was carried in the flat wagon attended by three horses and a plump old man.

As the huge man cracked the whip above his four horses he turned to Samuel. 'Herr Becker also asked me to give you a small gift to help with the tedium of the journey. You will find it behind you in the small storage compartment.'

Samuel lifted the lid of the rectangular box built into the space behind the front seat. A bottle of wine lay wrapped in a cloth.

'So, my friend now feels that I have need to find succour in the bottle.' His smile robbed the words of any insult.

'The good Councillor knows the journey to Molschleben will take us the better part of the day,' Heinz replied lightly. 'We must stop in Gotha to collect your wife's provisions, so Herr Becker thought you might enjoy it with some bread and cheese for your lunch. I am sure we can find a pleasant spot by a stream where the children can stretch their legs and ease their boredom.' The last was said with a wink to young Friedrich, who was helping Heinz keep a hold on the reins.

By a quarter after noon they had travelled to within a mile of Gotha. Samuel was pleased at the progress they had made, the warm summer making the journey much easier than he could have hoped. He recalled his first passage along this road with Heinz. In contrast to the weather ten months before, this day was almost balmy, with little breeze.

'A penny for your thoughts, Doctor Hahnemann.'

'I was thinking how Saxony never fails to delight me, regardless of the season or the place. Although,' Samuel's smile slipped a little, 'I'm not so sure that I should include our large towns in that praise; for all their fashion and culture they are little more than breeding grounds for disease.'

'Is that not a little harsh, doctor?' Heinz kept his question light, flashing a grin.

'Harsh? No, I would not call it harsh. I would call it honest. An honesty that is not recognised by enough people.'

'I'm sorry, I don't follow you.'

'People don't understand the most obvious facts. Show me one town where excrement is not left in the streets to breed its miasma? Where is there a system of drainage that can take waste and rubbish away so that it doesn't pose a threat to the delicate health of our children or the infirm? Or even where there is enough fresh drinking water available.'

Samuel turned to his friend. 'How many times have you witnessed ruinous epidemics that have swept through a town causing countless numbers of inhabitants to be carried away dead or dying?'

'But surely, the things you talk about are part of natural life.'

Samuel favoured Heinz with a bleak smile. 'That doesn't mean our lives should always be at the mercy of nature. I have spent most of my waking life trying to understand my profession. I am fearful that there is much that is not understood about the health of our people and the way we deal with it. I have constant battles with my colleagues over the inadequacies of bloodletting and purgatives to cure disease.' Samuel cast an involuntary glance behind him at the storage box where the bottle of wine still lay. 'Next time you see our friend Herr Becker, ask him to show you the file of articles that I have contributed to his paper on those very subjects.'

Without warning the coach bumped over a deep rut. Friedrich, dozing in the comfort of his father's embrace woke with a start. His bleary eyes regarded his father. 'Will we be stopping soon, father?'

Before Samuel could answer, Heinz pointed forward, his words directed at Friedrich. 'There's a pretty little glade only a few hundred yards ahead. A stream runs through it.' The huge man then turned to Samuel and said softly, 'Perhaps we could rest there and give the children a break from this tedium.'

'Thank you, that would be a good idea. My dear wife and the family have been very patient.'

'Your children are a credit to you. I cannot recall another group of youngsters so well-behaved, particularly a group so bursting with life and energy as your own.'

Again Samuel mused. 'That is another part of the puzzle, my friend.'

Heinz's face creased in confusion.

'Health is not something that is a God-given right. If we do not manage our health well, we can only expect illness, and, ultimately, death will reward our carelessness.'

'But how do we protect ourselves from the ravages of disease? Surely when our time has come there is little we can do to refuse our maker.'

Heinz studied the edge of the road, searching for the entrance to the small clearing.

'That is what many of my colleagues would have you think, so that they can persuade you to consume more of their medications than your system can possibly survive. 'No,' Samuel insisted, 'there is much that you can do.'

Heinz uttered a short cry of success and pointed his whip off to the side.

'This is the clearing I spoke of. I think the children will be safe to run off some energy here.'

Heinz guided the team of horses through a small gap in the side of the road to an idyllic grassed clearing. A line of trees flanked a small stream that flowed smoothly in the direction of Gotha.

Gratefully, the weary travellers climbed down from the carriage. Johanna handed young Caroline to Samuel, who was waiting at the door of the coach. Before stepping down herself, Johanna handed Heinz a basket, which he took with his free hand, the other clasping Herr Becker's bottle of wine to his chest.

Samuel sipped from a goblet while watching his wife and

children walk by the stream. The two older children were playing a game of blindman's buff between the trees and shrubs.

'I must remember to congratulate Herr Becker, this wine is excellent. Are you sure you will not share some with me?'

'Thank you, no. Wine is a pleasure, but I have to admit it quickly goes to my head and I would be happier delivering you and your family safely to Molschleben than have us all lying in a ditch by the side of the road.'

'Your integrity does you credit, sir.' Samuel said with approval.

'Earlier you remarked that our health is at risk from the garbage and shit left in our streets. So why don't our town's councillors do something about it?' Heinz sat up from where he reclined on the grass.

'There are many things that contribute to our well-being. Good hygiene among them.' Samuel smiled, watching Friedrich discover his sister hiding behind a fallen log. He clapped his hands. 'Well found, Friedrich,' he called out, 'Now see how well you can hide.'

The large man leaned across and poured some more wine into Samuel's goblet. 'Clearly you love your family very much.'

'They are my very reason for living,' replied Samuel. 'That is why I am so determined that they should be protected from our own stupidities.'

Exasperated, Heinz returned the cork to the bottle. 'Doctor, how can I ever understand if you keep on running away from your answer?'

'I am sorry,' Samuel said in good humour, 'I will try, I promise. Are you aware of the practice performed by midwives to shape the head of a newborn infant while it is still soft? Or that of squeezing out the breasts of newly born female children?'

The large man shook his head. 'I have to admit to little experience of children or the birthing habits of midwives.'

Samuel understood. 'Both practices are potentially very harmful, yet we allow them to continue under the supposed watchful eye of our doctors.' He sipped some of his wine before continuing. 'Do our parents then take their children out into the fresh air where their lungs and their bodies can develop? No. And why not? Because no-one counsels parents on what is right or wrong in the rearing of their children.'

Heinz looked at Samuel in surprise. 'Surely that is because the things you are suggesting are strange ideas that have no widespread support?'

'Not so strange and not so short of support, I can assure you,' Samuel replied. 'Only last year I translated a book from the French. Many of the ideas I'm talking about were already being shaped there, although I admit I added a few of my own.'

Samuel covered his smile by turning his attention to his children for a moment. 'For their entire lives,' Samuel waved in the direction of the game of hide and seek, 'I have hidden my children as best I can from the stupidities of our society. I have even shunned the opportunities of work in our cities to shield them from the diseases carried on the air. You asked about our lazy civic officials. They don't even try to see the germs breeding in the rubbish they have allowed to stink and befoul our lives.'

'You truly believe that is how much of our disease spreads?' Heinz asked, holding out the bottle of wine.

'I believe it emphatically,' Samuel nodded, 'and I will go one step further. I believe we are as guilty for ruining our own lives as Judas was of betraying Christ. Our children are indulged with foods that are better suited to keeping them quiet than building healthy bodies. Our women wear clothes that are designed to create pain and suffering. How can they even breathe when they have spent hours forcing their chests into a space designed to fit half the amount being shoved therein.'

Samuel banged his goblet down on the grass beside him, a small amount of wine sloshing over the side. His cheeks were slightly flushed, his voice raised a fraction. 'Believe me, if you want to live a long and healthy life you must lay the foundations as early as possible, preferably from the time of birth.'

'But what if you haven't done that?' The look on Heinz's face was solemn. 'Are you then condemned to a life of illness and misery?'

'No, it is never too late to change bad habits. Anyone will benefit from being aware of the things that do harm to their bodies and their well-being. But I also have a word of caution. As much as I believe in the value of fresh air and of the need to minimise our exposure to diseases, I do not believe that every person is the same or that their bodies will grow or develop in the same way. Some people are blessed with stronger systems. Some react differently to certain foodstuffs. Therefore the risks presented to our health by society and the pigheadedness of our doctors are compounded a thousandfold by our own complexities.'

'Then surely it is no wonder that so little is done. How can simple people be expected to comprehend the scope of your talk?'

Samuel sighed, nodding at the truth of his friend's remark. The flush faded from his cheeks. When he spoke again his voice was much calmer. 'It is not the fault of the people, Heinz, it is the fault of those charged with the responsibility of caring for them, or with the responsibility of creating a society that can embrace both the thinking and the practice. A person's diet is at the root of it, yet most of our doctors have never even seen a text dealing with the proper maintenance of diet.'

Heinz slowly climbed to his feet. 'Doctor, I would like to understand more. Perhaps you would be kind enough to continue my education on our journey. For now we should gather your family or we will not reach Molschleben before dark. And we still have to stop in Gotha.'

13

Even from sixty yards Samuel recognised his friend. Councillor Becker stood beside the first of the four open wagons crowded into the narrow street. The wagons were crammed with men, with bandages and crutches littered amongst them.

Samuel called out. 'My good friend, what evil resides in the midst of Gotha?'

'Fortunately the evil itself is not within Gotha,' Becker replied, his hands on his hips as he surveyed the misery. 'But that has not prevented the revolutionary's fingers from spreading the obscenity of their war. Fortunately the French are already teetering on the edge of destruction only six months after they took off their king's head.'

Becker reached out to the soldier closest to him, a bloodied bandanna wrapped around his head, the cloth tied with a rough knot at the back, his left eye completely covered. Barely visible through the dirt and grime was the light blue breeches and yellow striped uniform of Frederick's Saxe-Coburg contingent. 'According to this fellow, Prince Frederick has them on the ropes in northern France.'

Heinz pulled the horses to a stop a few yards short of the hospital wagon. The ears of his horses twitched nervously. On either side of the narrow street, gable roofs loomed over them. Beneath them, the cobbled tiles were littered with rubbish and excrement thrown from houses.

Samuel hurried across to Councillor Becker. The two men greeted each other with a firm handshake, their free hands grasping the other's arm.

'I see you have made the acquaintance of Gotha's toughest transport baron,' Becker teased. Without waiting for an answer he turned to the hospital wagon, his expression serious once more. 'These men have been sent home from the war to reclaim the Netherlands. They're perhaps some of the lucky ones who survived, but they will always carry the scars.'

Both men stepped back at a warning from the driver, who flicked his reins across three horses. Becker waved to the wounded man and then turned back to embrace Samuel.

'It is truly good to see you. Your family is well?'

Samuel nodded. 'A little weary from this tiresome travelling. I must thank you for arranging such excellent transport ... and the wine,' he remembered to add. 'I think I may have enjoyed one glass too many for lunch. I gave Heinz a lecture on the questionable ways of our medical fraternity.'

Becker clapped Samuel on the back. 'So why am I not surprised. Will you never change?'

'I suspect not. At least not until some of my brethren see the light and determine that their way is the wrong way.'

'I can see that my presses will continue to burn hot under the rhetoric from both sides. Only this week I received a letter from one of your colleagues in Hanover who had treated Klockenbring some time ago. His tone is decidedly chilled on the matter of your fee for curing the Minister for Police.'

'Still?'

'I am afraid so. Others have also published commentaries on your exploits. Reinhardt is writing a biography and has begun the most overt self-publicity.' The publisher chuckled. 'He has taken to writing letters to the editor in which he teases the readers with titbits. He claims to have recently asked the Bailiff of

Georgenthal, "how many lunatics does Hahnemann have in his asylum?" Apparently the magistrate's witty reply was: "One, and that is himself."'

Unexpectedly, Samuel broke into laughter. 'I shall have to buy a copy of his book when it is published. Perhaps I could get Reinhardt to sign a copy for my library.'

Becker waited for his friend's mirth to subside. 'Ah, yes, your library. I suspect that half of this load,' Herr Becker waved in the general direction of Heinz and the carriages, 'comprises books. How many have you published now?'

Samuel shrugged, embarrassment touching his cheeks. Playfully, his friend continued.

'I hear the number of pages has increased in the past three years by more than four and a half thousand. How much of that were your highly praised translations?' Herr Becker grasped Samuel's arm, shaking him gently. 'Speak up Samuel, I can't hear you.' Herr Becker smiled as Samuel shuffled in embarrassment. 'Of course everyone knows of Cullen's *Materia Medica*, that on its own would have been sufficient labour for most. Even Monro's two volumes would have exhausted other translators, not to mention your impressive work on that Italian's treatise on how to make wine. And all this whilst writing original works of your own.' Becker shook his head, pleasure resonating in his voice at the growing look of discomfort on Samuel's face.

'Enough of your depraved humour, Herr Becker. This is my work and yet you would poke fun at it?' The smile on Samuel's face was now as broad as his protagonist.

'But I have not finished.' Becker's face took on a serious expression. 'You have not allowed me to congratulate you on your election to the Academy of Science of Mainz to add to the fame you had already gained when elected to The Leipzig Economical Society. They do you incredible honour, and it is my privilege to consider such an illustrious and recognised person my friend.'

'Enough, you have truly embarrassed me now.'

With a broad smile and a gentle nod, Becker acknowledged

his victory. 'So tell me, my humble friend, what of your plans now? I have written to my colleague in Hamburg as you requested, but I am still uncertain why you have taken one of the good Frau Karstädt's modern houses in Molschleben rather than travelling directly to Hamburg.'

'As you have so cruelly pointed out, I suspect that my writing has suffered in the past few months while I have focused my energies on curing the Minister for Police.'

'Suffered ...' Herr Becker spluttered.

Samuel grinned, this time the humour his.

'Yes, it is time for me to again concentrate on my writing and my experiments. Of course these past months have been a blessing in some ways. The fee I am to receive from Klockenbring will enable the family to live in reasonable comfort for a time.'

'You still haven't been paid?'

'No, I understand there to be a problem with the man's finances, which have been in the hands of the court. He assures me that it is soon to be resolved and I shall have my money.'

'It must be particularly galling to be criticised for the fee you negotiated and yet not to have been paid,' observed Becker.

'Very, but I must believe that he will pay me, and have patience accordingly.'

'Considering he is cured, your patience should not have to be tested. But I suppose that is the way of the modern world. Were you able to do more in proving your Law of Similars?'

'With mercury you mean?'

Becker nodded. 'Didn't you tell me that Klockenbring had syphilis?'

Samuel hesitated. 'Yes, and I treated him accordingly, with doses of mercury, in the belief that the same response I induced on my own body would cause a peculiar counter-irritation in a syphilitic.' Samuel paused to wipe a hand across his forehead. 'It was no different to my earlier experiments, but I am still not sure that mercury was the single factor.'

Becker brushed Samuel's conservative response to one side. 'Come, you are too modest by half. And don't tell me that now, even with this latest success, you still don't propose to practice?'

Samuel considered the question for a moment, pursing his lips in thought. 'I think it is prudent of me to consider my position. You know me well enough to understand I cannot become one of the sheep. I must get some sense into my own mind, about the things I believe in.'

'I think I understand, but why hide in a village like Molschleben? Why not come back to civilisation?'

'There is much to be done, and it is far more practical for us to reside where the costs of living are lower. Molschleben also offers my children the fresh air they need.' With a hesitant smile Samuel paused before announcing, 'I am also pleased at the prospect of our sixth child.'

Becker thrust out his hand. 'My congratulations, sir, you made no mention in your letters. I am thrilled for you both.'

'Thank you, but we must be careful that we are not too premature in our celebrations. My wife has yet to reach the end of the second month. I will need to save all our pennies from now on; the costs of feeding and housing a family of eight is no small outlay, particularly when they have a breadwinner as contrary as theirs.' He smiled at his friend. 'I am delighted that we have had such an unexpected opportunity to talk, but I am conscious that my family still has two hours of travel in front of them and I cannot expect them to wait for me whilst I have a pleasant discourse with a good friend.'

Samuel carried a box of pots and pans to the back of the house where the modern kitchen was the object of rapt attention of Johanna. 'I insist you and your employee should stay the night, Heinz. We have room in this wonderful house and it is much too late for you to return to Gotha.'

Free of the last load, Samuel walked up to his wife and placed an arm tenderly around her shoulder. 'Are you all right, Elise? It has been a particularly long day for you.'

'I am fine. Stop fussing so. It is not the first time.'

'Do you think you will be happy here, for the birth of our

next child?'

Johanna raised an eyebrow and smiled at Heinz before turning back to her husband. 'So you will settle for a few months. Is that the confidence I should take from those words?'

'At least a few. I will need every bit of that time to prepare my next work.'

'Oh, and what pray tell will that work be?'

'I think I will write a lexicon, a dictionary for those people who need one the most — the apothecaries and the doctors. In it I will describe the ideal pharmacy of the future, where tinctures will be prepared from fresh, clean plant matter, where poisons would be kept under lock and key and where medicines would be prepared in such a manner that they would be guaranteed to be safe.'

Johanna regarded her husband with a weary smile. 'And when, pray tell, did you come up with this ... this ambitious idea?'

'I have been thinking about it for some time, but I have to say that this journey has been the catalyst.' Samuel turned to Heinz. 'Something you said crystallised the thought in my mind.'

Heinz regarded the doctor with surprise.

Samuel nodded in confirmation. 'I think you said something like, "how can simple people be expected to comprehend the scope of which you talk?" You do yourself a discredit, Heinz, but I understood the intent of your words. And you were right. How can I possibly expect people to understand the scope of my ideas unless I can frame them myself? The starting point must be an exhaustive work that proves my credentials as a chemist and a botanist; a lexicon that apothecaries and doctors can use and, by using, force them to question their current flawed methods.'

14

Samuel stood in front of his worktable. The top was littered with books and equipment for small experiments. At one end, a bunch of plant leaf had been left to wilt. Huge volumes lay open, leather bookmarks carefully laid across the pages. Steam poured from a glass beaker that sat over a small burner. Samuel worked with a mortar and pestle, a whitish powder filling the base of the stone bowl.

'What's in it, papa?' The young girl watched intently as Samuel ground the powder, the grains becoming finer by the moment. On her face a number of nasty eruptions spoiled her otherwise pretty countenance.

'Equal parts of sulphur and dry hepar sulphuris.'

'Hepar ... I'm sorry papa.'

'Hepar sulphuris. It is better known as powdered oyster shells.' Samuel's response was matter of fact, almost terse.

'Oyster shells? Like the oysters that come from the sea, papa?'

'Precisely. When I have crushed them to the finest powder they will be heated to form a paste. When it is finished I will paint the solution onto your face. The same with Friedrich and Wilhelmina.'

The girl looked at her father with wide eyes, her innocence, he could swear, designed to break down his censure. 'Why will you not paint it on Amalie and Caroline?' the young girl asked.

'Because, unlike my eldest daughter and her brother, they did as their mother and I told them.'

'But, papa, I didn't know that boy would pull my hair and then try to kiss me.' The young girl of ten stood defiantly, hands on hips. 'Anyway, it was horrible. I don't want any boy to kiss me again.' Her mouth quivered as she fought to prevent tears springing from her eyes.

Samuel smiled as he reached across to turn out the small white flame. When he turned back to face his eldest daughter the smile had gone, replaced by the same stern look he'd had on his face as he'd lectured his two eldest children. 'When I forbade you to play with the children in the village I did so with good reason, not because I wanted to punish you. I had reason to suspect that they suffered from milk crust and that if you were exposed to them you would also become infected.'

'But all we did was play a game of hide and seek. None of the others could find me, only that horrid boy.'

'Then it proves my fear was well-founded. Clearly the infection was very contagious and you are now suffering the same as that boy you seem to have taken such a dislike to.'

'Herr Braun, I urge you to consider the evidence. Two days ago my children were covered in sores; their faces in particular were unpleasant to behold. From the first application of the remedy they began to improve. I have kept them in quarantine since then and their symptoms are all but gone. Samuel lifted his hands in exasperation. 'That I don't practice should not be the reason for the other children to suffer, surely?'

Samuel sat in the drawing room of Mayor Braun's home, only a short distance from his own lodgings.

'Doctor Hahnemann, it is not up to me. I am simply the mayor of our delightful town,' replied Herr Braun. 'The fact that you mixed the medicine yourself, I suspect, will not be well received by the apothecary, Herr Schaefer.'

Samuel nodded. 'Sir, I assure you, I have no intention of setting up in practice in your beautiful village and I am more than prepared to explain that to Herr Schaefer, as well as Doctor Jurgen and Doctor Glockenwiel.'

'I must admit that I would be pleased for someone to find some permanent remedy to cure the confounded crust. My pair have been bed-ridden on and off for the past few weeks. All that Jurgen seems to have achieved is to increase the nagging of Frau Braun.' The mayor looked guiltily towards the closed door as if he expected the daunting frame of his good lady to come bursting through it, ear first.

Samuel smiled gently. 'My reputation as a chemist is well-known, Herr Braun. I am currently employed in writing a lexicon for use by apothecaries and am widely published on the subject. I have also earned a good reputation for conceiving many of the instruments that our apothecaries use in their administrations. I hope that Herr Schaefer will look upon me not as someone who is trying to deprive him of a living, but as someone who wishes to add to the nobility of providing relief to the sick.'

'You are right, Doctor Hahnemann. The suffering of our youngsters should be above all our other priorities. Heaven knows our lives are a struggle, without the added burden of sickness.'

Samuel nodded slowly, appearing to acknowledge the wisdom of the mayor. 'I endorse your comments wholeheartedly, and commend you for uttering them.'

Flattered, the mayor rubbed his hands together as he spoke. 'Then we should pay a visit to Herr Schaefer. By the way, have you enough of this ...? What did you call it?'

'Hepar sulphuris. A simple mixture, but an effective one.'

'Hepar sulphuris? Perhaps you would be good enough to remind me of the name when we visit Schaefer. I'm afraid some of these Greek words confuse me.'

'Latin, Herr Braun.'

'Eh?'

'The words, they are Latin.'

'The pleasure is mine, Doctor Hahnemann.' Schaefer shook Samuel's hand. 'I have seen your work. Your dissertation on the insolubility of certain metals and their oxides in caustic ammonia helped me resolve a particular dilemma of my own. I also have copies of both your Munro translation and the Cullen masterpiece.' The apothecary nodded towards the shelf behind him where the two massive texts sat side by side. Schaefer was a large man with a florid face and eyes that twinkled above round cheeks. He leaned across the counter and, with a conspirator's wink, spoke softly to Samuel. 'I am also something of a wine connoisseur, and I must admit I read with great pleasure and relief your instructions on how to determine whether wine has soured.' Schaefer leant back on his heels. 'I laughed uproariously when I learned that the Royal Prussian Chief Constable had used your piece to enact a law requiring all wine merchants to undertake the test.' He slapped the side of his leg. 'And that to do so they must purchase the necessary materials from a pharmacist.' The man's eyes were in the folds of his cheeks. 'My colleagues are four *gute groschen*, better off each time the constabulary threatens a merchant with an audit of his cellars. Pray tell you come bearing similar good news for the poor apothecaries of Saxony.'

Samuel smiled politely. 'Unfortunately we come with a request that will not make your fortune, Herr Schaefer, but one which I hope will prove beneficial to the village of Molschleben.'

Magnanimously, Schaefer spread his arms. 'How can I help? I would consider it a privilege to have assisted the work of a member of the Mainz Academy of Science.'

Samuel resisted the temptation to engage that particular gripe and concentrated on the matter at hand. 'I think I have found a treatment for the accursed milk scab that is threatening the happiness of our children. I have just finished treating my own, and it has cured them. I would like to make the same treatment available to the village, at no charge, of course.'

The light went from Schaefer's eyes for the briefest moment. Then a tight smile returned to the apothecary's face, his eyes hidden in the crease lines. 'Has this treatment been tested thoroughly, doctor?' A hint of suspicion clouded the question.

'Not to the extent that you perhaps mean. But the ingredients, I assure you, are innocent enough and readily found on your shelves.'

'So, pray tell, what are these ingredients that will supposedly cure milk scab?'

Samuel realised with a sudden flare of anger that the pharmacist's suspicion was tinged with sarcasm. He drew a deep breath. As he exhaled, a picture of Johanna jumped into his mind, her eyes flashing a warning.

'A simple tincture of sulphur and powdered oyster shell. I applied it as a paint to the sores of my own children. Even after the first application the eruptions were calmed. After two days there was no sign left that my children had suffered at all.'

Schaefer's eyebrows rose half an inch. His brown eyes searched Samuel's for a trick.

'Sulphur and oyster shell powder, you say?'

Samuel nodded, his wife's patient voice urging him to remain calm. With a grim smile, he wondered if he was finally learning how to play this game?

Schaefer inspected his shelves before reaching up and grasping a glass jar. The label on the front was unclear, although Samuel suspected it held sulphur. Satisfied, the portly pharmacist returned the jar before shifting his gaze lower, his eyes sweeping from side to side. Finally Schaefer turned back to face Samuel, the charade over.

He regarded Samuel with a raised eyebrow. 'My shelf stock seems to be a little short of shell powder, but that is no bother, I can have some delivered in a few days time.'

'Perhaps in the meantime you would allow me to provide you with some from a small stock I keep for experiments.'

Schaefer's left eyebrow rose even further. 'I hope, doctor, that you don't intend to dispense your own ...' Abruptly, he stopped before solemnly nodding his head. 'Er, yes, that would be satisfactory. I can always return your supply when I have replenished mine.'

For the first time, Samuel relaxed. Schaefer's right to dispense medicines was unequivocal, however the opportunity for profit existed now, not in a few days time.

'What of our good doctors?' the mayor interjected.

Samuel and Herr Schaefer turned at the question from Braun, forgotten by both of them in the midst of their mental stoush.

'Who will discuss with them this potential cure?' Braun continued. 'Surely without the good doctors we are unable to move forward. I am right, Doctor Hahnemann, that you have forsaken any intention to practice?'

Samuel relaxed completely as he watched the implication of the Mayor's words wash across Schaefer.

Colour flooded the pharmacist's cheeks, the Mayor's words resolving both his monopoly and his profit. 'If the good doctor is not intending to practice then we will have to ask Doctor Jurgen and Doctor Glockenwiel to consider their responses to Doctor Hahnemann's remedy. If they are agreeable then I am sure we can reach a mutually acceptable position on the dispensing of it, eh, doctor?'

Samuel walked through the front door of their lodgings to be met by his four eldest children, all seeking an embrace at the same time.

Henrietta was the first to gain her father's attention. 'Papa, when can we go outside to play? Friedrich won't stop teasing me and he doesn't play fair.'

'That is untrue.' Friedrich raised his voice over his sister's accusations. 'She is the one who always fights with me.'

'Both of you please be quiet. I know it is difficult to be cooped up all day. Perhaps tomorrow, after I have paid another visit to Herr Schaefer'.

Reluctantly the children left, their heads bowed as they glumly considered another day inside the house.

Samuel found Johanna in the kitchen surrounded by

ingredients for her weekly bake. Ignoring the flour dusted across her apron he enclosed his wife in a fond embrace, careful of her heavily swollen belly. Tiny beads of perspiration edged her hairline.

Wearily she smiled at her husband. 'To what do I owe such affection? It is not like you to risk your street clothes in this way.'

'I wanted to thank you, sweet Elise,' he said.

'Thank me for what? For making your favourite pie?'

'No, not for the pie.' Samuel cast a glance at the kitchen table where he could see the baked apple waiting to be enclosed in its shell of pastry. 'Although the pie confirms my good fortune.' Samuel's eyes gleamed. 'I want to thank you for your wise counsel today.'

'My counsel? I haven't laid eyes on you since breakfast. When was I supposed to have given you this wise counsel? And pray enlighten me on what good words I said.'

Quietly Samuel spoke into his wife's hair as she rested against him. 'I had a small victory today, Elise. I persuaded the apothecary of the wisdom of using my tincture for milk crust. He agreed to speak to the village's two doctors with me.

Samuel sniffed the warm scent of lavender rising from his wife. 'I have promised Herr Schaefer some of my supplies until he can order his own.'

Johanna pulled back from her husband to look him in the eyes. 'And the apothecary did not attack you for having these supplies? Did not feel threatened by you?'

'That is when your counsel came to my aid. Each time I started to get angry you reminded me to hold my tongue, to keep my patience. You were as clear in my mind then as you are standing in front of me now.'

Johanna smiled up at her husband. 'Thank goodness,' she whispered, 'there just might be hope for you yet, Samuel. There just might.'

15

Johanna's sobbing had drawn him from the small study downstairs. Samuel was in the middle of a complex drawing for a new apparatus. His detailed description was already written for inclusion in the lexicon.

As he climbed the stairs he heard another cry, this time muffled. The glow of his candle revealed the closed doors of the children's quarters towards the back of the house.

He opened the door to his bedroom. The sour stench of vomit reached his nostrils. He crossed to the bed, glancing at the window to reassure himself it was still open. He pulled his woollen gown tighter as a draft of bitterly cold air hit him.

'Are you all right, my love? Is there anything I can bring for you?'

The covers rippled slightly as Johanna shook her head.

'Are you warm enough?' Samuel persisted.

Again the blankets rippled in response.

Samuel looked at the basin on the floor where Johanna had just been sick. Much of the light supper she had shared with him before retiring had been returned.

'Are you still feeling nauseous?' This time the nod was followed by a cry of 'yes' as Johanna's head burst from the covers. She flung herself to the side of the bed. What was left of her supper found its way unerringly to the basin.

Samuel dipped a cloth into a small bowl of water, applying the compress to Johanna's mouth to wipe away a small drop of spittle. He returned the cloth to the bowl to freshen it before bringing it back to wipe her brow.

'I will get you some ipecac, that should ease the nausea, and perhaps a small glass of water.'

Johanna smiled weakly. Carefully Samuel collected the bowl at the side of the bed, his own stomach starting to churn from the contents. Will you be all right for a few moments?'

His wife's voice was weak. 'Is there something you can give me for these blessed legs, Samuel. They are again swollen.'

'This has not been a happy confinement for you has it, my sweet?' Not really expecting a reply, Samuel walked to the door, the bowl held gingerly in one hand, his candle in the other.

Samuel looked up as his wife pushed the door to his study open, a wan smile on her face. 'Do you feel better this morning, dear Elise?'

'A little. And what of you? Did you again work through the night?'

'Old habits are hard to break. I am sure that my brain works better at night, and this, I must admit, is becoming a taxing labour.' Samuel nodded at the pile of paper on his desk before laying the quill down. 'Had I known what I was getting myself into I suspect I might have sought counsel from some wise old man.' He smiled up at his wife, 'or an even wiser woman.'

Johanna laid a hand gently on her husband's shoulder. 'I don't feel particularly wise this morning. I suspect a male's hand in this, and before you make some vulgar comment, I am referring to the sex of the unborn infant not your virility.'

'Well, certainly your humour is brighter this morning.' Samuel patted his wife's hand. 'Has the swelling in your legs eased?'

'Yes, perhaps you should tell Herr Schaefer your secret remedy.'

'I suspect Schaefer has already made sufficient profit from

my ideas and suggestions. But we will see; if it suits my purpose then I will give it due consideration.' Samuel's smile was replaced by a more sober expression. 'I must admit I have changed my mind about Schaefer. My first reaction was that he was no different to all the others and that his only motivation was profit.' Samuel smiled at the surprise on Johanna's face. 'Oh don't get me wrong, I still think money is a very powerful lure for our good pharmacist but he has surprised me with his liberal thinking. He has an astute mind that grasps new ideas quickly.' Samuel glanced at the apparatus on the table. 'By the way, I did tell you that he will be visiting this afternoon?'

Johanna hid a smile behind her hand.

'I have asked him to give me his comments on this laboratory equipment I am working on. It is a nuisance not to have access to some of those bright students in Leipzig, but beggars can't be choosers.'

Johanna slapped her husband's shoulder. 'Sometimes, Samuel! Your arrogance will one day bring you undone. I can only hope that our second son does not inherit such an obnoxious trait.'

'You are convinced that we are to have a son?'

'And about time! Even I can become frustrated with a brood of girls.' A proud smile betraying her words.

'Herr Schaefer, it is good of you to come on such a foul afternoon.' As Samuel opened the front door a gust of wind threatened to send the pharmacist's hat flying across the thick layer of snow on the ground.

'It is my honour. I am not often accorded the privilege of mutual discourse with such a noted and respected chemist, not to mention such a renowned botanist as yourself. It would have taken more than a few inches of snow to deter me.'

Samuel took the apothecary's heavy topcoat and scarf and hung them on the rack beside the front door. Schaefer caught a glimpse of the coal fire blazing in the hearth of the living room and took a step towards the warmth.

'I have a small fire in my workroom, I am sure we will be comfortable there.' Samuel said taking the apothecary's arm.

'Oh, of course. Please lead the way.'

An elaborate structure dominated the table. At one end a burner sat beneath a beaker. The mixture it contained was a light grey. From the beaker, a copper coil extended to a test tube suspended above the table by a clamp attached to a metal stand. A steady drip of fluid fell from the end of the coil, splashing into half an inch of clear liquid in the bottom of the test tube. From the tube, a thin glass pipe rose no more than six inches before curving into a second beaker at the other end of the table.

'Herr Schaefer, I am sure I don't need to instruct you in the ways of distillation. Unfortunately many of the contraptions we use to distil even the smallest amount are large and unwieldy, making it hard for pharmacists to conduct some of their own experiments in the safety and warmth of the apothecary. I would welcome your comment, sir, on the structure you see on the table.' Samuel waved a hand at the apparatus while picking up a candle with the other.

Before Schaefer could reply, Samuel continued.

'I believe I have found a simple and inexpensive way to conduct such experiments, and even allow apothecaries with limited space to produce some of the medications that they currently purchase from their larger contemporaries. Allow me to show you how it works.' Samuel looked at his visitor who regarded him with a frosty stare. 'Is there something wrong, Herr Schaefer?'

'Good sir, I did not come here to have the most basic of chemistry lessons.' The apothecary stood with his hands on his hips, indignantly appraising Samuel. 'You do not need to instruct me on the workings of a still, and what I see on your table is nothing more nor less than that, a still.'

Surprised, Samuel looked at the apothecary. 'It certainly wasn't my intention to insult you.' A frown creased his brow. 'If I have offended, I apologise, my wife tells me that I have a very poor grasp of tact, but I assure you it is only my passion and enthusiasm that leads me to such insensitivity.' Samuel held his hands up. 'Truly, it is not the process that I am anxious to show you, but how it will figure in the extrapolation of my theory.'

Somewhat mollified, the apothecary folded his arms across his chest.

Samuel leant forward and dipped the flame from the candle to the second burner. He then moved in front of the first beaker, pointing to the greyish contents. 'As you slowly heat a mixture of different chemicals, the ones with the lowest boiling point boil off first, leaving the others behind.' Samuel pointed to the copper tube. 'The condenser cools the evaporated vapour, bringing it back to a liquid state.' Innocently Samuel looked up at the apothecary. 'With your interest in wine you would have seen such an operation to make brandy.'

'Sir, you test my patience.'

Samuel flapped his hands, his face blushing. 'Please, Herr Schaefer, forgive my clumsy tutorial.' Taking the man's silence as tacit approval Samuel moved to the very end of the table and picked up a bunch of dried leaves, some of which crumbled at his crude handling.

'For some time I have been observing the effects different medicinal substances have on the body. Even before I translated Cullen's *Materia Medica* I experimented with cinchona bark and discovered that it caused me to suffer all the symptoms usually associated with intermittent fever. If you have read my translation you would have seen the notations I made.' Without bothering to look for Schaefer's response Samuel continued. 'I have also experimented with other plant materials, and other substances, including mercury, which I believe cures syphilis by creating a peculiar counter-irritation in the body of the sufferer.'

'I have read the relevant passages, sir,' the apothecary said, 'and although I appreciate the logic I don't necessarily hold to your theory. What proof do you have? If I understood your commentary you only experimented on yourself and perhaps your family.'

'Which is more than my detractors have done.' Samuel blurted out angrily. 'Would you have us continue treating people with medicines that have had even less proof. Our doctors prescribe medicines, which you dispense willingly, that are often more suited to exacting revenge on someone for an imagined wrong than for their ability to actually cure.'

'How dare you. I take offence at your suggestion I would do anything to harm my fellow man. I may be, in your opinion, another greedy pharmacist but I can assure you that I am diligent in my energies to determine a more effective and compassionate response to the ills of our people.'

Samuel stared, stunned by the apothecary's outburst.

Schaefer continued. 'I am well aware of the shortcomings of our methods of treatment and I applaud you for having the fortitude to strike off in a new direction, but that does not give you the right to presume it is the correct one, or the only one.'

At last Samuel found his tongue. 'I assure you that it was not my intention to appear arrogant ...'

'Arrogant?' Schaefer spluttered. 'I suspect that arrogance is the root of your survival.' The apothecary spoke with less fire but stood firm, determined to make his point. 'I also am becoming disenchanted with the volumes of medicines that our doctors prescribe under the excuse of *contraria contraris*. Or, for that matter, that the prescription is too often based on the possibility it might be the right medicine.' Schaefer pursed his lips. 'I am comfortable in my life, sir, but I do not consider myself amongst the elite and see little point in dispensing medicines that do little to provide comfort or relief to those who take it. I would be very appreciative if you would remember that in any further discourse we may have.' Abruptly Schaefer turned on his heel and walked to the door of the small room.

'Herr Schaefer, please ... it was never my intention to question your integrity.' Samuel placed a hand on the sleeve of the apothecary. 'I would very much value your opinion on my theory, and to have the opportunity to debate it with someone of a like mind, or at least with someone who will not just throw my idea to the wolves without inspection.'

'For fifteen years I have deviated from what is considered the normal practice of medicine. Attending to my patients in the way the text books suggested was no different than taking out some kind of punitive revenge on the poor patient.'

'So what did you decide to do?' Schaefer took a sip from the glass of pale beer before replacing it on the small table. The two men sat opposite each other, a new log burning brightly in the hearth.

'I chose to abandon practicing. In all honesty I could not watch people suffer from unknown diseases and treat them with medicines that were equally unknown. To prescribe medicines because they were the best fit frightened me, as it should have frightened the poor sufferers.'

Schaefer appraised his recent nemesis with a smile. 'Perhaps our doctors should be grateful that their public adopts a fatalistic approach to these things.'

'An apt choice of words. Except that I had no wish to view myself as a murderer of my fellow man. If I didn't practice, then I couldn't be accused of adding to people's suffering. So I gave it away and concentrated my energies on my chemistry and my writing.'

'And experimenting on yourself.'

Samuel nodded. 'Yes, most definitely, but I was only driven to that decision after the birth of my first child.'

'I'm sorry doctor, why should the birth of your firstborn have such an effect?'

'I was confronted from the very earliest days of my daughter's life with the agonies that childhood sicknesses impress on all parents. Where was I to get help for her when at the very best our knowledge of these ailments rested on vague observations and hypothetical opinions?'

'And you believed you could correct that by experimenting on yourself?' A tinge of sarcasm crept into the apothecary's voice.

Blithely Samuel smiled. 'Of course.' His smile broadened. 'I am sure our wise God did not put us on this earth to be wiped out by our own physicians.'

Schaefer couldn't help himself. Laughter spilled from his lips just as he was about to take another sip of beer. He brushed the small drops from his tunic and then regarded the man sitting opposite, a smile still playing on his face. 'So how did you go about helping our God solve this dilemma?'

Samuel ignored the sarcasm. 'By observing how different medicines act on the perfectly healthy human body. I began by treating myself with minuscule amounts of medications such as cinchona bark, and observed what happened. From that I attempted to correlate their effect on my body or on those of my children and friends.'

'So you have been experimenting with others. I must admit that was something of a guess on my part.'

'Most assuredly, Herr Schaefer, but only ever with small dosages so that the effect could be reversed quickly if need be.'

'And did you have occasion to do so?'

'Yes, but never with any serious consequences. And what I learnt from it is intriguing.'

'How so?'

'What I set out to prove is that certain medicinal substances had effects on the body that mimicked certain illnesses, and that those substances could, in turn, be used to treat those particular illnesses.'

'And you are confident that you have proven that theory?'

'The truth is, no. Many of the substances I have tested have achieved what I set out to achieve. Unfortunately others have not. And until I can be truly assured of the soundness of my argument I must continue to experiment.'

Without warning the door to the drawing room burst open. Henrietta rushed in but came to an abrupt stop when she saw Schaefer. The young girl curtsied to the pharmacist and then turned to her father. 'Papa, quickly, mama needs you. I think she is having the baby.'

16

'Friedrich, please answer the door. Your mama is feeding the baby,' Samuel called out from his study where he was crushing a handful of dried leaves in his mortar. Again he heard the knock on the door. 'Friedrich, hurry, my hands are busy at the moment.'

'Yes, father, I'm going.' The pounding of feet echoed through the house as the young boy ran from the kitchen. For a moment there was silence, then a loud squeal. Putting the pestle to one side, Samuel turned to the door of his study just as a huge hand appeared. As the door swung open Samuel saw his son struggling valiantly in the arms of a giant.

'Heinz! What a wonderful surprise.' Samuel smiled as his son tried to prise himself out from the huge man's grip.

Heinz held the boy at arm's length while the youngster grasped for the big man's nose. 'You've grown in the past few months, master Friedrich, but still not quite enough to get the better of me,' Heinz said as he swung the boy down to the floor. He held out his right hand to Samuel, his left resting casually on top of the boy's head. Friedrich swung his arms uselessly.

'What brings you to Molschleben, my friend?'
'The giant chuckled. 'The truth is, you do.'
'I do?' Samuel lifted a quizzical eyebrow.
'Once again I have to offer my thanks.'

'Why? What did I do this time?'

'Herr Schaefer, doctor, the good apothecary of the town.'

'For once I agree with you.'

'I'm sorry ...' a look of confusion appeared on the giant's face.

'Nothing, nothing, ignore me, I was being facetious. Please don't let me interrupt your story, what has Herr Schaefer to do with this welcome visit of yours?'

'I have gained a contract with some of the village merchants to haul their supplies from Gotha. Herr Schaefer recommended my name to them.' Now it was the giant's turn to raise an eyebrow at Samuel. 'My anonymous referee to the rescue again.'

Samuel scratched his head. 'I had forgotten. Herr Schaefer asked me a month ago if there was someone I could recommend in Gotha. Naturally I gave him your name, you being the most reliable of a bad bunch.' Samuel placed an arm on the huge man's sleeve. 'Come, I will make you some tea. Frau Hahnemann is upstairs feeding the newborn.'

'Congratulations once again. That's six, if my memory serves me.'

'Your memory serves you well. Young Friedrich has a young brother to whom he can teach bad habits.' Standing beside the giant the young boy began to protest until he saw the smile on his father's face.

'I am delighted that your business is doing well, Heinz, although it provides me with something of a dilemma.' The two men sat at the kitchen table, a pot of weak tea between them.

'Why so?'

'I have decided that I need to move my family for their improved welfare and to ease my finances. I am earning some money from my writing but it is a slow and precarious livelihood and it is unlikely that I will see any money from the first part of the Lexicon for at least a year.' Samuel looked around the kitchen. 'Unhappily, we are drawing too much from the fee I earned from Herr Klockenbring. This house is costing me a fortune and our living expenses, even here in the country, are sending me to the poorhouse.' A frown creased Samuel's forehead. 'I have decided to move the family to Pyrmont.'

'The resort town?'

'The very one. Have you ever been there?'

The giant shook his head. 'No, but I am told that it is very beautiful. Some call it the summer residence of princes.'

'I have heard the same, and I have also been told that there is a lucrative opportunity for me there if I desire to return to practicing.'

'And do you?' Surprise etched the big man's face.

'Bluntly, no. But I think it is time that I took my duties as a parent a little more seriously.'

'From what I have observed, your children are a credit to you. They are also the healthiest children I have seen anywhere in Saxony, thanks to your principles.'

'For a man who has never seen Pyrmont, or too much fifty miles either side of Gotha for that matter, that is quite a claim,' Samuel gently chided Heinz.

'You know what I mean, and I do not withdraw one word. I feel desolate that I am unable to help. I have committed to three new contracts and the rosters my lady has drawn up will be the ruin of my health, although not my bank account.'

Samuel clapped the big man on the shoulder. 'And you deserve every pfennig. Do not feel bad because of your good fortune. You have worked hard for it. There is a man in the village who I understand takes such charters and I am afraid I can't delay. If I am to take this job I need to be in Pyrmont before the start of the season.'

'Are we agreed then sir?'

The surly driver nodded his head. 'Aye, we're agreed, but I've been taken. You're the winner from this arrangement, no question. It will take the better part of two weeks to get you there and me back, if you are so insistent on travelling a lousy ten miles a day. We could do much more and that's a fact.'

Samuel ignored the man's grumbles. The price was a fair one according to Heinz. 'If you don't want the job, sir, I can find another who will be glad of the money. I will not put my wife with a two month old baby through any more inconvenience. Ten miles a day it will be. Is that understood?'

'Aye, it's understood. And I'll be here for an early start. Be sure you're ready too.'

Samuel turned on his heel, the last remark unnecessary. Unless the man changed his attitude Samuel could see a very unpleasant trip looming. Yet he had checked everywhere. There was not another coach and driver to be had this side of Georgenthal or south of Gottingen who could have him and his family in Pyrmont before the job offer was withdrawn.

17

'Father why can't I sit up the front?'

Samuel observed the driver, the expression on the man's face no different than the day before. *You are definitely the most objectionable man in all Molschleben,* Samuel thought to himself.

'There is barely room for the few belongings we are taking. As it is, most of the furniture will have to follow in a month or so.' Samuel looked at the boxes of books and personal clothes that had been tied to the top of the carriage. The space beside the driver was equally cluttered. He placed an arm around his son. 'I'm afraid we will all need to find some comfort within the carriage.' Finally he called to the driver, 'We should aim to make our first stop the village of Mulhausen. I have arranged for accommodation.'

With a sneer the driver looked down on Samuel. 'I thought you insisted on ten miles doctor? Mulhausen is at least twelve.'

'Sir, I am sure we will get on a great deal better if you could leave your unpleasantness here in Molschleben to await your return.'

Samuel hugged Friedrich to him. 'Climb aboard, son, I think your mother will need all our help today. Perhaps you and Henrietta would look after the two young ones whilst your mother nurses baby Ernst.'

Solemnly Friedrich nodded to his father and climbed aboard. For the first hour Samuel nursed his new son, his wife dozing against his shoulder. The miracle in his arms gave him enormous pleasure and great pride but he worried about the health of his beloved Elise. Her confinement had left her weakened. Samuel had prescribed a tonic but was scathing of his own inadequacy to do more.

Across the carriage his two eldest children were amusing their younger siblings. The smallest, Caroline, sat happily on Henrietta's knee immersed in a game of "I spy". As the game flagged, Samuel prompted a new round picking the cows in the meadow as the object of his "I spy". With a grin, Friedrich whispered into his youngest sister's ear.

Wide-eyed, Caroline looked out the window of the carriage, her excitement growing as she saw them. 'Cows, papa! There! In the grass.' Samuel nodded his head as the young girl jumped up and down on her sister's knee. 'My turn, my turn. I spy somefin' beginnin' wif "t".' The letter flattened by the young girl's tongue.

'Now what could that be?' Samuel asked, watching the trees on the side of the road flash past as the carriage kept up a lively clip. In his arms the baby gurgled as the other children took up his prompt, taking their time to go through all the things they could see beginning with "t". Finally five year-old Amalie lifted her eyes from the book on her knee.

'It's obvious.' Amalie's eyebrows arched disdainfully. 'Trees, "t" for trees.'

Crestfallen at her sister's pronouncement, Caroline's bottom lip pursed.

Samuel hid his smile, nodding his head seriously. 'You know the rules, Caroline, its Amalie's turn.'

Her lip still pursed, the young girl turned to Amalie, waiting for her sister to utter a letter. Now that she was the centre of attention, Amalie dropped her eyes to the book in her lap, affecting no further interest.

'Papa, not fair. Amalie won't play,' Caroline called out to her father.

Samuel regarded his third daughter. 'Amalie, are you playing or reading?' The small girl raised her eyes to look at her father. 'It's a silly game.'

'Then don't spoil it for everyone else,' Samuel rebuked his daughter before turning to Caroline. 'You may have Amalie's turn, Caroline. Apparently she doesn't want to play.'

Samuel settled back into his seat. The swaying of the carriage caused Johanna's head to bounce gently against his shoulder. He braced himself with his foot against the door, trying to ease the jarring for his wife. In his arms, the baby gurgled contentedly. They would need to stop in an hour or so to enable Johanna to feed him, but for the moment Samuel was content, grateful that his children gave him little cause for chastisement. He looked with pride at the newest of them, painfully aware that Johanna had often blamed herself for the presence of so many females. He had given up counting how many times he had reassured her that he cared only that they were all healthy.

'He is so beautiful' Johanna said softly, her cheek still lying against his shoulder. 'I am so pleased God saw fit to present us with such a handsome child. He will be a good son to you, just like Friedrich.' Johanna reached over to gently move the light blanket away from her son's face. 'Perhaps he will follow in his father's footsteps and become a famous physician.'

'I would not wish such a future on my worst enemy.' Samuel smiled into his wife's eyes. 'Not even Robespierre himself.'

The coachman stopped without warning. Samuel craned his neck through the window, his view blocked by the coachman's legs swinging down from behind the horses.

'What is happening?' he yelled.

'How should I know? I'm going to check.'

Cursing the man's rudeness Samuel opened the door, a glance at Johanna warning her and the children to stay in the coach.

The carriage had stopped on a gentle incline where both sides of the road were edged by a low bank. Ahead, the cutting rose until it reached the height of a man's shoulder. Samuel walked up the slope until he came level with the lead horses, where their driver was standing with hands on hips. Twenty yards ahead, a large tree had given up its tenuous hold on the left bank and had crashed across the road, blocking it in both directions.

'Well, doctor, have you any clever suggestions?'

Samuel bridled at the tone but bit his tongue. 'Is there another road?' he asked.

'Back about two miles.'

'How far are we from Mulhausen?'

'Another hour would've seen us there.'

'And if we double back?'

'At least three.'

Samuel stroked his chin. If they doubled back it would be dark by the time they reached the village. Yet to clear the tree would be almost impossible for the two of them.

'Have you equipment we could use to clear the tree?' Samuel asked.

'Yeah, I've an axe, which you're welcome to. But don't expect me to give yer any help. I ain't gettin' paid to do no manual labour. I sez we back up and let some other poor sap clear the mess.' Without another word the man turned on his heel and strode back to the coach, leaving Samuel with little choice but to follow.

'He is an accursed man,' Samuel whispered to Johanna. 'I will bear his surliness until we get to Gottingen then I shall pay him out and find another with a more civil tongue in his head.'

They had travelled for nearly an hour to reach the detour to Mulhausen. Every few minutes Samuel checked his timepiece until Johanna had been forced to lay her hand over his. Robbed of his distraction, he tapped the fingers of his right hand impatiently on his knee until finally, unable to hold back, he pulled the watch out again and flipped it open. 'We still have an hour's travelling ahead of us, Johanna. I am afraid the children will be exhausted.'

'There is nothing to be done for it. Please try to be patient.'

Alarmed at the look of exhaustion on his wife's face, Samuel reached across to take the infant from her arms. Johanna smiled weakly at him. 'Stop fussing, Samuel Hahnemann, I am fine. Do you hear me? Fine. Perhaps you would be good enough to think of some amusement to keep the children occupied.'

From above, came a crack of the whip as the carriage reached a level stretch of ground. During the day the coachman had urged his horses on at every opportunity, cursing the deep ruts left by the harsh winter. In some places the melting snow had washed away the surface of the road leaving it treacherous. Samuel braced his foot against the door, loath to instruct the driver to cut his pace if it would gain them time. The children had also found handholds to stop from being thrown around. With his free hand Samuel pulled Johanna closer to him, her hands occupied with the baby.

The hollow pounding of hooves on timber dragged Samuel's eyes to the carriage window. A bridge flashed past, offering a glimpse of a roiling stream swollen from the mountains. Then they started to climb.

Trees lined the roadside closest to him, a cutting on the other side grew higher and higher until he could see nothing else. The coachman gave no sign of slackening his pace as the road beneath them continued as smooth as any they had travelled all day.

Friedrich had a broad smile on his face as he hung onto the door with one hand and his sister's coat with the other. Samuel was sure the boy would have whistled and whooped if he had not thought his father would caution him. Unlike their brother, the girls wore grim faces, the eyes of the two youngest, shut tight. Johanna looked at her husband, a note of concern creeping into her eyes.

Samuel said, 'I don't think his surliness has yet turned to recklessness. I will caution him if he goes any faster.' Johanna turned her attention back to young Ernst.

Above their heads the coachman returned the flask to the

pocket of his woollen overcoat, a grin etched on his face.

'Please, Samuel, speak to him. The appeal of this speed seems to have palled even with our Friedrich,' Johanna said, her eyes on their eldest son.

Samuel glanced at Friedrich. The boy's earlier joy had been replaced by a tight grimace, the effort of hanging on while holding Caroline clearly taking its toll.

Grasping the spar between the door and window Samuel pushed his head through the opening. The wind and cold slashed at his face making his eyes stream. The side of the cutting flashed past his head.

'Enough, sir! We are being shaken to pieces inside here,' Samuel yelled in the direction of the driver.

Above him the driver cracked his whip, urging the horses faster, the road ahead a clear run for a hundred yards or more.

'Sir, I insist. You will cause someone an injury.'

'What was that?' Again the whip cracked overhead. 'Fraid I can't hear you, doctor.'

'I said, enough, we wish to reach the village in one piece.'

'Sorry, doc, I can't hear you, the noise up here is deafenin'.'

With laughter ringing in his ears, Samuel withdrew his head into the carriage. He grasped both sides of the door as he stood and thrust his head through the larger opening above, ignoring the entreaties behind him from Johanna.

'I insist, sir! Slow this coach immediately. You are risking all our lives.' Terrified, he watched the coachman draw back his whip and lash it across the four horses, spurring them to even greater speed.

A hand grasped the back of his coat. 'Samuel, please, you are frightening me. Please come back inside. The madman will surely kill us, but you put yourself at even more risk. Please.' As Samuel turned to reassure his wife he caught a glimpse of a small boulder on the side of the road. The lead horses were just abreast of it as the coachman again lifted his whip, cracking it above the ears of the lead pair.

'Watch it, you **fool**!' Samuel screamed at the driver. 'There is a rock.' Samuel pointed. 'You fool, you cannot miss it.'

Helplessly he watched the coach close the distance until the left wheel clipped the rock causing the carriage to lurch violently. Samuel's head slammed into the top of the door, opening up a nasty gash on his forehead. Blood streamed into his eyes as he fell back, sprawling across Johanna. Around them, the carriage swayed wildly, threatening to turn on its side as the wheel climbed into thin air. Unable to grab a handhold, Samuel slid across the floor, the screams of his wife and children filling his head. The carriage crashed back to earth, the front wheel bounced once, twice. Samuel was trapped in a tangle of legs. He tried to haul himself to his knees but lost his balance as the carriage swayed violently from one side of the road to the other. Above him, rocks and mud flashed by the window, the carriage swinging dangerously close to them until, with a violent rending of timber, the earth wall tore a hole in the side of the carriage only inches from Friedrich's head. The carriage lurched away from the cutting, its right wheels no longer on the ground.

Bodies and limbs flew in every direction. The carriage crashed onto its side. The terrified horses dragged the coach along the road for a distance before the shaft tore loose from the body and the crazed horses raced away.

As the wreck settled, a single wheel continued to turn lazily in the late afternoon sun.

18

'Aaaaghhhhh'.

The scream tore at Samuel's heart. Sweat broke out on his brow as he tried to move his legs. A moan came from behind him. He squinted through the dust and gloom. A tangle of limbs lay around him. His head ached from the blow against the door. He touched his brow, his fingers came away sticky with blood.

'Johanna? Are you all right?' he called out softly. 'Johanna, please answer me.'

Around him the sound of crying grew louder.

'Friedrich? Can you hear me?'

A groan came from behind him.

Samuel felt the softness of an arm under his body. 'Friedrich, are you all right?'

'I think so, papa. I'm not sure.' The boy's voice was on the edge of tears.

'Caroline, what about you? Can you hear me, Caroline?'

'Yes, papa.' Her voice was muffled. Then the young girl began sobbing.

'Caroline, listen to me.' Samuel's voice was sharp. 'Are you hurt? Did you scream?'

The young girl's sobs became a snuffle. 'I'm frightened, papa, I can't move! My leg, it hurts. It hurts so much.'

Tears sprang to Samuel's eyes at the wretchedness of his daughter's plea. 'Stay calm, I will help you, just stay calm.'

Samuel's eyes adjusted to the light and began to pick out the colours of his family's clothes. Above his head he could just make out the handle of the door. He reached up for it but his fingers failed to make the target by the width of a nail.

'I have to try and open the door. I am going to see if I can free my legs. Children, do you understand?'

The sobs from beneath him grew louder.

'Amalie? Wilhelmina?' There was no answer. Oh my dear God, prayed Samuel, please let them be all right.

Samuel moved his left foot, feeling the firmness of timber under it. His right leg remained trapped. Slowly he pushed down with his left, pausing to see if he had trapped anyone's arm. Again he reached up, his fingers brushing the handle. Applying more weight to his foot he gained another few inches until his fingers grasped the handle.

'Johanna, can you hear me? Please answer me?'

Finally: 'Yes, I banged my head. I'm all right. But Ernst?' The panic in Johanna's voice was clear to all.

'I'm trying to open the door. Please stay calm.' Samuel twisted the handle and pushed. The door flew open only to crash back to its frame. Cursing, Samuel again pushed the door with every ounce of strength he could muster. It flew open, teetering at the top of its arc before crashing onto the side of the coach.

Samuel was breathing heavily. 'Friedrich, can you climb onto my shoulders? You will have to help me get the rest of the family out so that I can free my leg.'

The boy reached out and put his arms around Samuel's neck. 'I will try but I think my leg is also trapped.'

'It may be caught under someone. Please, everyone, if you feel Friedrich move his leg, see if you can help him free it.'

It was Amalie who cried out, lifting herself off the side of the carriage where she was lying. Samuel breathed a sigh of relief at the sound of his daughter's voice.

'Now, Friedrich, see if you can get onto my shoulders and

climb through the carriage door. Do you think you can do that?'

'Yes, father, I will try.'

Slowly Friedrich hauled himself up onto his father's shoulders until his head poked through the doorway.

'Can you see the driver, Friedrich?'

For a moment there was silence, his family awaiting the answer as eagerly as he.

'No. He may be trapped too.'

Cautiously, Friedrich lifted himself from his father's shoulders and swung a leg over the side of the carriage until he was completely outside.

'I'm going to pass Amalie out to you. Is there a way for you to climb down to the ground?'

'I think so. I can climb over the driver's seat.'

'Good boy. Can you help Amalie down that way?'

'Yes, papa.'

'All right. When I pass Amalie out I want the two of you to climb down and then wait for me?'

'Yes, papa.'

Samuel reached out and plucked his third daughter from between the limbs of the others. He held her in his arms a moment and kissed the tears from her eyelids. Quietly he explained what he wanted her to do while pointing to Friedrich, whose head and shoulders were visible through the doorway above them.

He called out to his son, who reached down and grasped the little girl's arms, careful not to lose his balance while he helped pull her out.

'Now, Friedrich, very carefully, help Amalie climb down.'

Samuel cursed the driver as the pair disappeared from his view.

The young boy's voice floated in through the carriage doorway. 'We're safe, father. Amalie's down here with me. Do you want me to climb back?'

'Wait a moment.' Samuel turned, grateful to see Johanna clasping the baby to her breast her eyes staring straight ahead.

Henrietta sat on the side of the carriage next to her. Caroline lay unconscious, her leg twisted at an awkward angle, his own leg trapped under the girl.

'Dearest Elise,' Samuel spoke quietly but firmly, 'Caroline may have a broken leg. I can't free myself until everyone is out. Can you help?'

For a moment Johanna stared straight ahead, then a tear appeared in her eye and rolled down her cheek.

'Johanna, please I need your help.'

She turned to Samuel, tears coursing down her face. She nodded without a word.

'Henrietta, please take the baby,' Samuel said to his eldest child.

The young girl turned to her mother, her hands outstretched to take young Ernst. Without speaking, Johanna handed the bundle across to her daughter, wrapping the blanket tightly around the baby as she did so.

'Johanna, I will help you climb through the door and then pass Ernst to you. Do you understand?' Mutely, Johanna nodded. She stood, grasping the sides of the door. Samuel wrapped his arms around his wife's hips and pushed her through the opening until she lay sprawling on the side of the coach.

Samuel passed the baby up, grateful to feel the warmth of his cheek, the only part visible in the swaddling.

'Friedrich, can you hear me?'

'Yes, papa.'

'If your mother passes Ernst to you, can you reach him?'

'I think so. If I climb onto the driver's seat I can.'

'Good boy. Johanna?'

Samuel couldn't see his wife nod. An agonising moment passed, broken by a shout from his oldest son.

'I have Ernst, papa. What shall I do now?'

'Hold him, Friedrich, hold him close.'

He turned to his oldest daughter. 'Your turn, my sweet. Like your mother, all right?'

Henrietta nodded and stood up. She cast a nervous glance

at her sister lying unconscious against the door of the upturned coach.

Samuel lifted her, his arms around her hips, pushing her out through the door.

Finally he turned to Caroline, whose eyelids were fluttering. Gently he touched her leg. A moan escaped from the girl's lips. Samuel reached down with his arms and tried to lift her.

Caroline screamed, the ear shattering noise cut short as she passed out. Samuel scooped Caroline into his arms and painfully stretched his trapped leg. A cramping pain lanced up into his groin. Samuel winced, trying to ignore it. He stood and called out to Henrietta and Johanna, who had both remained on the side of the upturned coach.

Henrietta answered. 'I am here, papa. But something is wrong with mother. She won't speak.' Samuel heard the tears in Henrietta's voice, his own despair for his wife making him choke back his own tears.

'I am going to pass Caroline up to you. Can you lie her on the side of the coach? Please be careful, she has broken her leg.'

'I will try, papa, I will try.'

Samuel watched his oldest daughter reach through the doorway and grasp Caroline around the chest, pulling her none too gently through the opening. 'Careful, my sweet,' he whispered.

'I'm trying, papa. I'm trying not to hurt her any more.' Tears poured from the young girl's eyes.

'Yes, I know you are, my sweet.' Tears poured down his own face as he waited for Caroline to disappear, then he dragged himself up through the opening.

He looked down through the suspension of the carriage. Ernst lay quietly in Friedrich's arms, Amalie and Wilhelmina stood by their brother's side. With a sense of disquiet, Samuel jumped, landing a few feet from where the small group stood. Another sharp lance of pain shot through his leg. He turned back to the overturned coach and reached up to where Johanna held their youngest daughter. Gently she passed the girl down.

Johanna looked at Friedrich and his small bundle. Her two sons shimmered in a stream of tears.

Samuel held his wife's hand. The pair were seated in the front row of the small church.

'It is for the best, my beloved Elise. Who can know what his life might have been like if he had survived? That he lived for even three days was a miracle.'

The tiny coffin rested forlornly in front of the altar, the kindly priest prepared to welcome all of them into his church in their time of grief. Caroline had been unable to come, the pain in her leg forcing Samuel to give her a few drops of laudanum.

'It was my fault.' Johanna's eyes filled with tears, the words spoken between her sobs. 'I didn't hold him tightly enough. I saw his head when I picked him up from the floor of that wretched coach,' Johanna sobbed as she relived the painful memory. 'If only I had held him closer.'

PART THREE

KÖNIGSLUTTER, 1799

19

'Frau Haller, I assure you that you only need take the amount I prescribed. Because Doctor Keller insists on prescribing horse tablets does not make the practice obligatory. It certainly doesn't for me.'

Frau Haller inspected the small phial in her hand. She peeked at Samuel from under her bonnet. 'Please don't misunderstand me, Doctor Hahnemann, we are grateful that you treat us and don't charge for your medicine but it seems so, so strange.'

'I don't see what is strange about it. Haven't your family responded to my treatment? It is these others that are fools ...' Samuel bit off the retort, as Frau Haller's hand flew to her mouth.

'Please, trust me,' Samuel said, his anger under control. 'I assure you, you have no need to ingest huge quantities of medicine for your ailment. Within a few days it will be gone.'

Samuel smiled wearily as the gentle lady hurriedly crossed to the door. Samuel caught up to her. 'Good day, Frau Haller. Remember: six drops before your evening meal, then a further six drops when you rise for breakfast.'

The woman nodded as she slipped gratefully through the door.

Samuel heard the passage door open behind him. Johanna stood in the doorway to the kitchen.

'Samuel, I insist that you take a break. You have already seen five patients this morning. I am warning you, your lunch will spoil if it is forced to sit on the stove another minute.'

Before Samuel could answer, Johanna turned and left. Sadly he walked back to the room where he received his patients.

How he wished the light would return to her eyes. Johanna hadn't been the same since the death of little Ernst. Samuel cursed, 'Damn that man!'

That the driver had died from internal bleeding gave Samuel no comfort or consolation for the shattered health of his dearest Elise. Frederika was a blessed child, but Samuel suspected their new baby would never replace Johanna's beloved Ernst. Perhaps if their seventh had been another boy? Perhaps.

For the thousandth time he rued the offer of a place at Pyrmont. Had he not wavered to the lure of financial gain Ernst might still be alive.

Impatiently, Samuel got to his feet and smacked his clenched fist against his leg. 'It is more than four years, for the love of God, two of them here in Königslutter. How much longer will you drive yourself insane with guilt?'

Samuel walked out of his study into the small sitting area set up for the use of his patients. He tidied the sitting area and returned to his study to put away his notes. Then he would do as his dear wife bid.

The knock was barely loud enough to catch his ear. He stopped mid-stride, wondering if he had mistaken the noise for something else. The second knock was firmer but still barely loud enough to disturb him. He crossed to the outer door and threw it open before the timid creature could flee.

The girl in the doorway stood no more than five feet tall, a heavy cloak struggled to conceal her slimness. Unlike her figure her raven hair was revealed, the hood pulled back carelessly from her face. A clear brow sloped to a pert nose, the porcelain white of her skin delicately set off her beauty. A scar, a jagged crescent perhaps an inch long, ran from the corner of her eye to the high plane of her cheekbone. And her eyes were the most brilliant green Samuel had ever seen.

Samuel stared at the intriguing woman before remembering his manners. 'I'm sorry, Fraulein, my rooms are closed, you will have to come back tomorrow.'

'Doctor Hahnemann?' The question hesitant.

'Yes!'

'Sir, I beg of you, please let me speak. I have walked here from near Helmstedt to seek your help.'

'I'm sorry but I have work that needs my attention. All my patients appreciate that I have to have rules to follow, otherwise nothing would ever get done.'

'I appreciate there must be onerous demands on your time, but I beg of you don't send me away without allowing me five minutes. Five minutes please, Doctor Hahnemann, then I will willingly leave you in peace.'

Samuel reassessed the young woman. She truly was just a slip of a girl, with no outward sign of illness or hurt, unless you considered the small scar.

'Fraulein, what can I offer in five ...?'

'Frau, Frau Wendt.'

'I'm sorry, madam.' Samuel blushed softly. 'I did not presume you old enough to be married.'

'My husband of four years was killed twelve months ago in the service of Prince Frederick.'

'I'm truly sorry, Frau Wendt, but I cannot alter my program on every compassionate tale I am told.' The woman's green eyes locked on his, determination etched into them. Sensing her resolve Samuel took a deep breath. 'All right, five minutes, but then I must take my leave and attend to my family and my other duties.'

Relief flooded Frau Wendt's face. Samuel sensed she was fighting to hold back tears. He pointed her towards the study.

'Doctor, I will come to the point without delay.' Frau Wendt brushed the back of her hand across her eyes as she sat in the visitor's chair. 'There is an outbreak of sickness near Helmstedt. I fear that my four children may have been exposed to it so I have isolated them from the rest of the children in the village.'

'You have done what?' Samuel's voice rose with incredulity.

Frau Wendt blinked in surprise. 'Isolated them, sir. Isn't that what you would have done?'

'Well, yes, I believe so. But where did you determine the rules of quarantine? And, in particular, how they apply to a fever?'

The woman forgot her tears for the moment. 'In the first instance, on the battlefield of Valmy.'

'Valmy? The defeat of Brunswick?'

The young woman nodded.

'But how, for Heaven's sake, would you encounter disease during a bloody battle?' Samuel scratched his head, dumbfounded.

'There had been an outbreak of smallpox in a village near where the French engaged the duke's army. Before the battle, Brunswick sent his surgeons to inspect the extent of the outbreak. I was a novice. Our order had been sent to care for the sick.

'You were sent with ... but I still don't understand, a novice does not normally learn the rules of quarantine. Most doctors don't truly understand them.' Samuel could not keep the surprise from his voice.

'For that I am grateful to my late husband, who was one of Brunswick's surgeons'

'I'm sorry?' Samuel gave up any pretence at patience. 'In one breath you tell me you are a novice, in the next a widow. Which is it?'

Frau Wendt bit her lip. 'Doctor Hahnemann, the story of my life is of no importance, but you asked when I had first seen the pox and, I am sure you would agree, the first time stays firmly pressed in your mind.'

Samuel recovered his composure and considered the woman with interest. 'Yes, it does. As a young woman I'm sure you found it particularly disturbing.'

The slight woman returned his gaze steadily. 'No more so

than the other ills that the nuns taught me to care for.'

Samuel nodded slowly. 'What do you believe is the malady that afflicts the children of Helmstedt?'

'I hope that it is scarlet fever.'

'You hope?' Surprise coloured Samuel's question.

'Yes. Again I saw the symptoms in France.'

'But you are not sure?'

'No, I am not. There has been talk of smallpox in the vicinity.'

'Smallpox?'

'Apparently a small outbreak occurred in a village a few miles from ours, on the road to Magdeburg.'

'I have heard nothing of this. How could we allow a disaster to brew on our doorstep without some sort of warning or intelligence? Please, carry on. Have you seen the symptoms in your own village?'

'Not as I understand the symptoms, no. But a friend asked me to look at her child.' The young woman saw the question in Samuel's eyes before he could ask it. 'My neighbours know of my training with the nuns. We have no doctor in our village, sir. When I visited the child she had a rash that had tiny bumps under the skin. The rash had already spread from the face to the neck, but the area around the mouth was clear. When I pressed the rash it blanched white.'

'The rash was red of course?'

Frau Wendt crossed her arms. 'Of course. Surely that question was unnecessary'

Samuel ignored the rebuke. 'And the child's throat?'

'The throat was also reddened, and the poor child's temperature was over 100. Oh, and the glands were badly swollen.'

'Did you see white specks on the tongue or at the back of the throat?'

'Yellowish more than white. The tongue was becoming furred.'

Samuel considered the information a while then said, 'Your

observations are very precise, madam, you do your training credit.' Frau Wendt's stiffened arms relaxed a fraction at the unexpected compliment. 'What symptoms have your own children shown?'

'When I left them this morning one of the twins had already developed a rash, like a flush from too much time in the sun.'

'And there was no sign in the other three?' Samuel's smile was gentle, the bristle gone from his demeanour.

Frau Wendt shook her head and dropped her hands to her lap.

'What age are your children?'

'I had the twins last, a boy and a girl.' A tear glistened in the woman's eye. She wiped it with the back of her hand. 'My eldest daughter is nearly five, her brother is three,' Frau Wendt corrected herself with a smile. 'Three and a half. He is very determined that I shouldn't forget the half. The twins are nearly two. Their father was killed before they could celebrate their first birthday.'

'How do you think the child contracted the disease? The neighbour's child?'

Frau Wendt nodded. 'I had asked her to care for the twins whilst I cared for another child who had broken an arm. When I returned I noticed that the girl had a slight rash on her throat, but I paid scant attention to it, what with the twins crying for their dinner and all.'

Madam, I am impressed with your resourcefulness. The people of your village are indeed fortunate to have you. I presume you fear an outbreak of this disease.'

'Yes, my neighbour's daughter is welcome in many homes because of her generous and caring manner.' A smile appeared briefly on the woman's lips. 'Perhaps in this case the good folk may not be so appreciative of her generosity.'

Samuel returned the smile, delighting in the woman's quick wit. 'Why did you come to me, Frau Wendt? Doctor Keller has been here much longer than I.'

'I had heard your name from my husband, when we lived

in Magdeburg. He once attended a lecture at the hospital given by Professor Christian Hufeland, the Chair of Medicine at the University of Jena. My husband told me later what had occurred. Apparently a doctor asked him a question about you.' A blush crept up the throat of the beautiful woman. 'It was not very complimentary.'

'They very rarely are?' Samuel smiled.

'According to my husband, Professor Hufeland praised your writings. He called you a refreshing catalyst of change, and that the medical world needed more like you, people who were prepared to challenge methods that were doomed to the past'

'I am grateful to Christian. We do not agree on all things and I am sure he sometimes thinks I go too far. But he never refuses to publish me when I am trying to establish a new theory. You have read his journal?'

Frau Wendt smiled. 'Yes, many issues, although not since my husband died.' She smiled sadly. 'I must be honest and admit to having been nervous about approaching you. I was ready to flee from your door if I could find the excuse.'

'Madam, I assure you I am more than approachable.' Samuel playfully added, 'Perhaps I'm a little crusty when I'm pining for my lunch.' He got to his feet. 'I am confident that what you describe is scarlet fever, but if there is smallpox in the vicinity I think it prudent that we take no chances. I will arrange a carriage. This afternoon I will return with you to your village and inspect the children.'

'Did you isolate your twin from the rest, Frau Wendt? Where?' Samuel followed the wave of the woman's arm around the single room. His heart ached at the memory of his family's similar struggle in Stotteritz.

'The best I could hope for was to keep them from the other children in the village. I have kept their eating and drinking utensils separate from my own and have washed everything thoroughly in hot water.'

'I am impressed, Frau Wendt. I have pushed for these

concepts until I'm blue in the face. I'm delighted to find someone with the same common sense.'

Frau Wendt blushed at the praise, covering her embarrassment by turning to collect something from the kitchen table where her eldest daughter was sitting. The three youngest children were confined to their cots.

Samuel held the back of his hand to the young girl's forehead. 'There doesn't appear to be any fever. Nor does there appear to be any fever in the other two. Yet the twin is well advanced in her incubation. I have no doubt that she has scarlet fever, but your other children intrigue me. The second twin and your son are flushed around the neck but neither seems to have come down with the fever.' Samuel turned to the eldest. 'As for your eldest, she has absolutely no signs of the disease. Absolutely none!' Samuel smiled at the small girl. 'What is your name?'

'Madeleine,' the little girl said sheepishly, a hesitant smile brightening her face.

'What a pretty name. I have five little girls of my own. The oldest is now grown to a beautiful girl of fifteen, the youngest is only one.'

'What are their names?'

'The eldest is Henrietta and the youngest is Frederika. Between them are Wilhelmina, Amalie and Caroline.' As Samuel talked he inspected the girl's throat and pressed the glands at the side of her neck.

'You have no boys?' Frau Wendt asked.

'Yes, I do. My second eldest is a boy. His name is Friedrich. I'm afraid he has a hard life, always having to compete with five girls for his mother's and father's attention.' Samuel smiled as the little girl laughed.

'It puzzles me that Madeleine shows no symptoms of the disease at all. Does she have some special diet that distinguishes her from the other children?'

Frau Wendt shook her head slowly. 'She likes carrots more than the others.' Madeleine and her mother exchanged smiles. 'Apart from that I can think of nothing.'

'Has she had some other complaint that the smaller children did not suffer from?'

'No, nothing that comes to mind, not in the past few months. The smaller children have had sniffles, colds, but Madeleine also caught them.'

'Mama,' the young girl pulled at her mother's dress, 'do my sore fingers count?'

Samuel asked, 'What was the matter with your fingers?'

'They were very sore and swollen.'

Samuel looked to Frau Wendt for more information.

'The joints in her fingers became inflamed when she was playing a few days ago. I wasn't sure what it could be. She complained of catching her fingers when she fell, but there were also scratches and I was fearful a nettle might have stung her. I gave her some belladonna, and I've been giving her small amounts each day since. The swelling and the inflammation have almost gone.'

'How many days?'

'Why?' Frau Wendt appeared bemused. 'The inflammation is all but gone and it was caused, I am sure, by the girl's fall.'

'How many days?'

Frau Wendt bit back her surprise at Samuel's abrupt manner. 'At least three, perhaps four.'

'Before you saw the symptoms emerging in the twin?'

'Yes, well before.'

'In Königslutter you said that you had read Hufeland's journal?' Samuel raised an eyebrow at the beautiful woman. Frau Wendt nodded. 'Did you ever read any of my articles or essays?'

'Yes, quite a number. I have also been fortunate to see some copies of Herr Becker's *Der Anzeiger*.'

'Madam, I had no idea your reading of my work had been so extensive.'

Frau Wendt crossed to a small cupboard. She returned to the table with two heavy volumes. 'It is, in part, thanks to your writings that I am able to help so many of my neighbours.'

Samuel opened the front cover of the first book. He knew

the words off by heart. The first edition of his *Pharmaceutical Lexicon* had been well received and was already considered an essential standard reference. The reviews, particularly the review in Hufeland's *Journal of Pharmacy*, had been glowing. With a pang of guilt he thought back to his desk where the final pages of the latest edition waited his attention.

Beneath the Lexicon was a copy of Cullen's *Materia Medica*.

Samuel turned the pages of the thick volume, pleased to find them well-thumbed. He looked up. In an article I wrote a year or two back I discussed the curative powers of drugs.' He waved a hand in dismissal. 'The lengthy title of it was somewhat pretentious, but the essence of what I now believe was written there.'

'I have some memory of your theories, Doctor Hahnemann,' Frau Wendt shrugged her shoulders.

'I have a suspicion that the belladonna you have been giving Madeleine may have something to do with the reason why she has not contracted the scarlet fever.'

'The belladonna? But belladonna has never been used to treat scarlet fever.'

'If we are to truly understand the effect that drugs or medicines have on the sick we must have the patience to first experiment with the drug on the human body when it is at it's full power.'

'What you say is familiar to me. My husband and I often discussed your papers. If I recall correctly, your proposition was that an effective remedy will incite a kind of illness peculiar to itself.' Samuel waited as Frau Wendt searched her memory for the words. 'And the more acute or marked the illness that resulted, the more effective the medicine.'

'Again, I must compliment your recall. I argued that we should treat the disease to be cured with a remedy able to stimulate another, artificially produced, disease, as similar as possible to the one being treated. In this way the treated disease would be cured. Or *similia similibus*.'

'Likes with likes?

'Correct, Frau Wendt. And in your daughter's case I am hopeful that she may be proof of the efficacy of belladonna in a way that has not yet been considered.'

'To treat scarlet fever?'

'Perhaps in both treating it and preventing it.' Samuel took a deep breath, fearful to take the step he desired. 'I ...'

'Can it harm the children, Doctor Hahnemann?'

Samuel's heart was pounding. 'I'm not sure I understand your question.

'In the past I have given the children belladonna to treat inflammation. If they are given it to prevent scarlet fever, can it harm them?'

'I ... I don't think ...' Samuel searched for the right words as doubt crept into Frau Wendt's eyes. 'I can assure you that the belladonna will have no ill-effect if it is used to treat scarlet fever in your children. My hesitation comes from my reluctance to experiment on others. '

Frau Wendt searched Samuel's eyes for a sign of doubt or hesitation. 'Sir, I don't think your confidence is born from recklessness. There is nothing else that I can think of that has set Madeleine apart. The only thing is the belladonna.' She placed an arm around her daughter's shoulders and hugged the girl to her. 'I am prepared to trust you, Doctor Hahnemann.'

Samuel narrowed his eyes. 'I assume you still have the belladonna you were using to treat Madeleine?' Frau Wendt nodded. 'If I treat Madeleine and the two children who are still to show all the outward signs, it will be as a prophylactic. The twin I will treat to see if it will also cure. But be aware, madam, that I will only give them the minutest part of a single grain.'

'Please don't treat me as a fool. How could such a small amount prevent anything, particularly something as virulent as scarlet fever?'

'I assure you I am not trifling with your intelligence. If you will trust me to treat them with belladonna then please trust me to prescribe the amounts that I believe will work.'

The cough woke Samuel from his uneasy sleep. A small lamp burned next to the stove, giving off a dusty light. From where he sat in the rocking chair he couldn't see the cots of the twins. The two eldest children shared a small bed near the kitchen table. A rough curtain had been pulled to give some privacy to the bed where Frau Wendt had retired, exhausted. She must have woken some time during the night and covered him with a blanket. In the dim light he opened his fob watch, surprised that it was already past one in the morning. He stretched his legs, the movement causing the heavy volume of Cullen's *Medica* to slide forward. He grasped it from under the blanket to stop it from crashing to the floor.

Quietly, Samuel pulled the blanket to one side and lowered the book to the floor and crossed the room to where the four children slept. Leaning over the twin with scarlet fever, he placed the back of his hand on the child's forehead. It still burned but, fortunately, for the moment, the child slept. He turned to the second twin and again placed his hand on the child's forehead. As far as he could tell there was no change, there was certainly no temperature. After checking the temperatures of the other two children he returned to the rocking chair and pulled the blanket around him, grateful for the mild night.

Samuel woke with a start. His eyes flew open, unsure what had awakened him. Frau Wendt sat at the kitchen table holding one of the twins. In her hand was a small bottle.

Discretely, Samuel coughed. Frau Wendt turned in her chair, a gentle smile on her lips. Samuel pushed the blanket to one side and looked at his watch. It was close to five in the morning. He stood and crossed to Frau Wendt obtusely pleased to see that the child was the sick twin.

'Is there any change in the others?' His whisper was answered with a hesitant shake of the widow's head.

Samuel walked over to the small lamp, turned the wick up a fraction and then crossed to the male twin. Again there was no sign of a temperature, and the flush he could see in the light was no worse than it had been in the afternoon. His inspections of the others failed to show any sign of the fever.

'There is no sign as yet. Perhaps in another twelve hours or so,' Samuel whispered as he sat down at the kitchen table. He placed a hand on the brow of the small child in the widow's arms. The temperature was still high and the rash had deepened in its colour. 'Frau Wendt, I must go back to my home and make sure my family is safe. I can only pray that the carriage driver had the sense to do as I asked and explained the situation to my wife. When I have finished with my patients this morning I will come back to see what change there has been.'

'Doctor Hahnemann ... please! I can come to Königslutter tomorrow and tell you what progress there has been. You have already done more than could be expected.' Frau Wendt hesitated. 'I am fearful that I am going to have to seek your further kindness and allow me to pay you when I have the funds.'

'We will worry about that another day. As for you coming to Königslutter, I will not hear of it. It is important that your children be kept in isolation, and I think, madam, that you are the only one who we can trust to do that.' Samuel smiled.

'But how will you get home?'

'The same way you did on your first visit to me. I shall walk.'

20

Over Samuel's shoulder the day's light was just starting to show in the pre-dawn. A line of trees stood vaguely silhouetted against the flat line of the earth. He was already a mile from Frau Wendt's lodgings and estimated he had three more to reach Königslutter. Another hour, he guessed, just in time for breakfast and a lecture from Johanna. He quickened his step a half-smile on his lips.

'Who goes there?'

Samuel's heart jumped at the barked command. His head snapped to the left, to where the voice came from.

'Who's that?' Samuel stammered.

A shadow loomed in front of him, followed by a second. In the darkness he could make out the shape of two horses.

'You have five seconds to answer my question or I will shoot.'

Samuel imagined the muzzle of a pistol pointing at him, but in the dark he wasn't sure. 'I'm Doctor Hahnemann. I have been visiting a patient in a village near Helmstedt.' Samuel's heart was racing.

'The truth man or I will put this ball between your eyes.'

'That is the truth. I'm a doctor from Königslutter.' Samuel pointed a thumb over his shoulder. 'There has been an outbreak of scarlet fever, possibly smallpox, in the village where I have been.'

'The pox? Are you sure?'

'No, but that is why I am forced to travel at this time of the morning. I need to be sure that there is no danger to the other villages. The spread of scarlet fever will be devastating.'

'I understand, sir.' A tone of respect entered the man's voice.

The dawn was starting to throw a pale light across the horses. Above them Samuel could make out a rounded helmet, a tall crest rising above it. His heart slowed. 'I have answered your question, sir. Why do you deem it necessary to frighten the daylights out of a man going about his lawful business?'

'I'm sorry, doctor. We are with the fifth regiment of mounted Jägers detailed to locate a band of deserters who fled during the retreat from the Rhine.'

As the light strengthened, Samuel could make out the dragoon uniform and white breeches of the German regiments of the Austrian army. The green comb on the helmet and the green facings and insignia on the man's uniform confirmed his identification.

'Where were these men seen, Captain,' Samuel asked.

'On the road from Brunswick. Apparently they were travelling east. We spent last night in Königslutter. We believe they may be heading for Berlin, where they can disappear into some bolt hole.'

'And you say there has been no further sighting?'

'So far, none.'

'Then, if I am free to go, I wish you luck with your search. It is still an hour's walk for me and I suspect I have a worried wife and family to report to.'

'Take care, Doctor Hahnemann, keep your eyes sharp. These men are desperate and looking for vulnerable targets.'

'I presume you have reason for frightening the children and me half to death?' Johanna blocked his entry to their home, arms folded across her bosom. 'As if it isn't enough that you should stay out the entire night, but you do so when we are awakened from our slumbers by the entire Austrian army searching for thieves and murderers who threatened to rape all the women in Königslutter and kill all the children.'

'Frau Hahnemann, I swear you exaggerate.' Samuel's eyes were wide in mock surprise. 'I met two of your so-called entire army on my return from Helmstedt. They are still out there searching for the deserters. It is my opinion that the deserters have got more brains than to be caught in Königslutter, where they would be unable to hide from the prying eyes of our neighbours. As for my absence, I have already offered my most abject and loving apology. I sent a message back with the coachman. Did he not deliver it?'

Johanna continued to stare. 'Yes, but he made no mention of you staying at the home of that calculating vixen.'

'She is not a calculating anything, Johanna.' Samuel raised his eyes to the sky, the reason for his unwelcome homecoming now clear. 'She is a distressed mother whose children have scarlet fever, at best. At worst we may be faced with an outbreak of smallpox.'

'Smallpox? You have been into a home with smallpox, and now you expect to be allowed to spread that death amongst your very own loved ones?' Johanna's horror was heartfelt.

Samuel reached out a hand to pat her arm but she immediately snatched it away.

'Don't touch me if you come bearing the plague.'

'It is not the plague. One of the children has scarlet fever. Several more in the village have also come down with it. Frau Wendt correctly recognised the symptoms, but had heard rumours of an outbreak of smallpox and wished to be sure. She was right to do so. If there were an outbreak of smallpox nearby I would want to know so that we could take steps to deal with it.'

'How can you deal with smallpox?' Johanna asked, her tone incredulous.

'Quarantine is one thing we can do. But enough of that, I

bear tremendously exciting news, Johanna.' Samuel paused and looked around. 'Come, let us continue this inside, all we are doing is giving the neighbours something to gossip about.'

Reluctantly Johanna stood to one side as Samuel walked into the house. 'I am parched after my walk. Do you have any objections if I draw myself a glass of water, or perhaps there is some of that delicious lemonade you made?'

'Don't you try to sweet-talk me; I tell you it won't wash. I still want to know what you and that ... that woman could find to talk about all night.'

Samuel ignored the irate look on his wife's face. 'This afternoon I must return to Frau Wendt's lodgings and check her children. By accident we may have found a means to treat scarlet fever.'

Johanna folded her arms across her chest. 'Then you might like to share that good news with Doctor Keller.'

Samuel tried to read the expression on her face. 'What does Doctor Keller have to do with any of this?'

'He came visiting yesterday afternoon looking for you. Apparently Frau Haller told him you had said he was no better than a horse doctor. He was seeking your blood, sir, I can assure you of that.'

'A horse doctor? Why would I have called Doctor Keller a horse doctor in front of Frau Haller? Samuel's mind swept back to the previous morning. *Was that only yesterday?*

The memory of escorting Frau Haller to the door jumped to mind.

'Prescribing horse tablets ... that's what I said to the damned woman.' Samuel threw his hands into the air. 'I said something about Keller prescribing horse tablets, for goodness sake. I was referring to his medicine not his practice.'

'Doctor Keller I can assure you I did not refer to you as a horse doctor.' I wouldn't be so disparaging to that profession, Samuel thought to himself.

Clear of his patients, Samuel had walked into town. His

intention had been to spread the news amongst the apothecaries and doctors, of the outbreak of scarlet fever around Helmstedt, and the possibility that there was smallpox about. He got no further than the first pharmacy, where a small group of doctors were gathered. Amongst them Samuel spied the portly figure of Doctor Keller.

'You rise above your station, Hahnemann.' Keller stood toe to toe with Samuel, a thick finger prodding him in the chest. 'I am sure I speak on behalf of my colleagues.' Keller turned his head briefly to the group, emboldened by the nods and grunts of support. 'You have the temerity to insult us in front of the good people of this town and expect us to say nothing? Well I can assure you we will have none of it.'

'My comments to Frau Haller were innocent ...'

'Sir, your comments to Frau Haller are of little consequence.' Keller once more prodded Samuel in the chest. 'Your constant and unsparing criticism of us is there for the entire world to behold in your writings.' Keller paused for a moment to allow the murmur of support from his colleagues to grow louder. 'Who are you to tell us what to do? To slander our good work! My father was a doctor before me, his father before him. My family has served the town of Königslutter faithfully for the past seventy-five years. You have been here no time at all and yet your arrogance allows you to defame us?'

'Defame you? How? By telling the truth?' Samuel pushed Keller's finger away with an angry swipe of his arm.

'To you, sir. The truth as you see it.' A second voice took up the argument while Keller stood open-mouthed at Samuel's aggression.

Samuel turned at this new attack, recognising the red-faced, gout-ridden Doctor Andress, with whom he had shared a number of civil discussions at the pharmacy. Andress stepped up. 'As Keller says, our colleagues and our predecessors have successfully treated patients for decades. Every one of us has a degree to prove our diligence to our oath, not to mention years of experience in caring for the sick and the infirm.'

'You call that caring, Doctor Andress? I call it cruelty. Caring is seeking ways to make sure your patients regain their health, not to just fill your pockets.'

'Now you go too far, Hahnemann.' A third doctor had joined the fray, a semi-retired doctor in his late fifties who had relinquished much of his practice to the aspiring Andress. 'In my entire life I have cured as many patients as I have lost. And I'm proud of it, sir. I don't need your fancy new ideas to deal with my patients.' He turned to his willing audience. 'The latest, I see, is that Doctor Hahnemann now considers himself a town planner.' The retired doctor turned back to Samuel. 'Am I not right, Hahnemann?'

Angrily Samuel choked back a reply, determined not to give the foolish doctor further ammunition.

'Did I not see your name,' the man continued, 'next to an article extolling the destruction of the old quarters of towns to improve hygiene, to rid the cities of the airless lanes where poverty dwells? Is it your intention, sir, to rid the cities of the air or the poor?' His audience dutifully laughed.

Encouraged, the man continued his attack, paying no attention to the steel that had crept into Samuel's eyes. 'He goes even further, telling our esteemed town councillors they should be levelling the embankments that surround our towns, to protect them, to allow the air, or is it the poor, to escape.'

Again the doctor's audience laughed at Samuel's expense, egging the man on. 'And wait there is more. Next we should drain the marshes and then lay out new suburbs for the comfort, I presume, of the poor that he has evicted from their homes.' Doctor Andress looked around his audience, his arms spread in expectation of his victory.

Samuel's reply was laced with venom. 'Unless someone has been quoting me, good doctor, the article you refer to was in fact written up in a small book I wrote seven years ago. Perhaps that sums up your own lack of currency, if you have only just read it.' Samuel stared at the doctor, whose smile was slowly turning to a sneer as Samuel's rejoinder sank in.

Samuel turned to the others. None of the group was prepared to meet his eyes. 'I came into town to give you a warning. Now I can see there is little point because none of you are prepared to listen. But be aware! Scarlet fever and smallpox are once again on the rampage. In a village nearby I have just treated four infants for scarlet fever and the rumour is that smallpox is blowing on the same wind.'

Samuel turned on his heel and strode away in disgust, leaving the gathering of doctors open-mouthed at his warning.

'There has been no change?'

'None, Doctor Hahnemann. Madeleine has been helping with the youngest ones and she has shown no sign.' Frau Wendt selected her words carefully. 'The twin appears to be improved, her temperature has dropped to a hundred. It had been as high as a hundred and one.'

'What of the rash?'

'At this time there has been no change, but the early signs on the other twin have disappeared.'

'Completely?'

'As far as I can tell, yes.'

'I must admit I am quietly pleased. It is only a couple of hours shy of twenty-four since the first dosage. We should give them another dose now, and then another at this same time tomorrow.'

'Have you warned the other doctors, as you had planned?'

Samuel nodded. 'I went to see them this morning. Unfortunately they were in no mood to listen to someone who they consider a quack and a troublemaker.'

'You are not a troublemaker but a man of considerable vision. It is a pity that there aren't more doctors prepared to make some contribution to the improvement of medical knowledge and understanding, rather than just criticising those that do.' Colour crept into Frau Wendt's cheeks as she spoke.

'Thank you for your confidence. Now I must return to Königslutter and pay some attention to the next edition of the *Lexicon*, which I fear has been badly neglected. I will try to return at this same time tomorrow to check the children's progress.'

21

The house in Königslutter stood on a wide street, a small garden added tranquillity to the front. The entrance was blocked by two large wagons. A youth sat on the box seat perched atop the second wagon. There was no sign of a driver for the first.

Samuel paid his coachman and bid him a good afternoon. He tipped his hat to the youngster on the wagon as he opened the gate to his home.

'Johanna, I am home,' Samuel called out, surprised when none of the children came rushing to meet him. He pushed the kitchen door open. Johanna and his five older children were seated around the kitchen table. At the head of the table the baby, Frederika, gurgled contentedly in the arms of Heinz. Samuel's face broke into a grin at the sight of his old friend nursing the child.

'Heinz, what a wonderful surprise after all these years. Now I understand why there are wagons outs ...' Samuel paused, the grin on his face slipping as the glum faces around him registered. 'What is wrong? Why does everyone look so depressed?'

Heinz reached out his huge paw to shake hands with Samuel, the baby nestled in the crook of his left arm. 'Your good wife will have to tell you the whole story, Doctor Hahnemann,'

Heinz replied, 'I arrived as the men were leaving, although I can attest to their anger.'

'Their anger?' Samuel's eyes widened. He turned to his wife. 'Who was angry, Johanna? Why should anyone be angry with you?'

'Not me, Samuel.' Johanna wiped a tear from the corner of her eye. 'They were not angry with me, they were angry with you.'

'Angry with me? Who were these ...' Samuel paused to stroke his chin; his next words were menacingly quiet. 'The town's doctors?'

Johanna shook her head. 'No, Samuel, not the doctors, the apothecaries, a delegation of apothecaries. They wanted to see you, to deliver an ultimatum.'

'An ultimatum about what?'

'That you stop dispensing your own medications or they will bring an action against you.'

'The doctors are behind this, Heinz, mark my words.' Samuel stared at the glass of pilsener in front of him.

Johanna sent the children to help the giant's stepson tend the horses. An invitation to join the Hahnemann's for dinner had been gratefully accepted but the giant had declined an offer of a bed, preferring that he and his wife's youngster camp with the horses and wagons next to a nearby stream.

Over drinks, Samuel continued his attack, anger colouring every word. 'Their jealousy of my success grows with each year we stay in this godforsaken town. Yesterday I tried to warn the fools of an outbreak of scarlet fever and to give them a possible treatment.'

'You have found a cure for scarlet fever?' Heinz was incredulous.

Samuel slumped back in his chair, a rueful grin twitching at the corner of his mouth. He lifted a hand in a dismissive gesture. 'Perhaps ... I'm sorry, sometimes my anger and my mouth seem to be on a collision course.' Samuel saw the look of confusion cross the big man's face. 'Perhaps a cure,' he conceded. 'I am treating a family in a village near Helmstedt, where there is scarlet fever. The treatment I have prescribed seems to be keeping three of the children free of the symptoms. The child who has the affliction has become no worse.'

'And what, pray tell, is this possible cure?'

Samuel stroked his chin, the smile on his face becoming broader by the minute. 'I think it would be wiser for me to keep that information to myself for the moment, Heinz. But perhaps in the morning you would be happy to take me to the village so I can visit the family and see what progress has been made. Then we will see whether my so-called miracle is working.'

'It would be my pleasure. I have to wait until the day after tomorrow to pick up the freight we are taking to Gotha. May I ask what you intend to do about the apothecaries and their threat?'

'I think I shall wait until I see the outcome of tomorrow's visit to Frau Wendt. There is no doubt that Königslutter is in the path of the fever. Within the next few days I am sure we will be seeing cases here. 'Who knows, if my miracle cure works I might finish up being the most popular doctor in Königslutter.'

The following morning three anxious mothers were waiting outside Samuel's rooms. Each of them complained that their children were running high fevers and were covered in a red rash. Samuel gave them strict instructions to return to their homes and isolate the sick children from the rest of the family. He promised that he would visit them as soon as his day surgery was complete.

During the morning, another two women appeared on his doorstep with the same tale. Forsaking lunch, Samuel went out and visited each of the five families and confirmed that the children were indeed afflicted with scarlet fever. He gave instructions for their care and the importance of keeping them quarantined from others in the household. He instructed the mothers on cleaning their eating and cooking utensils in boiling water and to ensure that none of the family ate from those utensils used by the infected child. He told each family that he would return later that evening with the necessary medicines.

It was after three in the afternoon when he and Heinz left Königslutter.

The small house where Frau Wendt rented her room was separated from the rest of the hamlet by several hundred yards and sat on a crossroads that intersected the wide expanse of fields. Storm clouds were gathering on the horizon as Heinz pulled the four horses to a stop.

'I fear we will be getting wet on our return.' Heinz punched a thumb over his shoulder at the dark clouds.

Samuel studied the gathering clouds. 'I won't be long, Heinz. It will only take a few minutes to check on the progress of the children. Frau Wendt is an extremely practical lady who does not need me to interfere. If everything is well then we can return to Königslutter poste haste and I can start treating the outbreak there.' Samuel climbed down from the wagon. 'Do you mind waiting here for me, Heinz, I think it would be quicker if I do this on my own.'

'I shall take cover in that copse of trees.' Heinz pointed to a stand of trees fifty yards past the house.

Samuel crossed the road noting that the curtains had been drawn across the two windows of the downstairs room. He approached the door and knocked twice, waiting patiently for Frau Wendt to open the door.

A short moment passed. Samuel lifted his hand to knock again, his ears pricked for any noise from inside the room. Samuel rapped more loudly on the door. The hairs on the back of his neck prickled at the thought of some disaster with the belladonna. No, it was impossible, the belladonna could do no damage, not in the small amounts he was administering. Anxiously, he reached for the door handle and twisted.

A flicker of surprise grabbed at his stomach as the door was wrenched open, catching Samuel off balance. A hand grasped his arm and pulled him into the room, sending him crashing to the floor. A whirl of images raced through his mind: a pair of rough cotton trousers over heavy boots; a musket propped against the wall; the children cowering in a corner of the room; an unkempt figure dressed in infantry grey holding a pistol over them, his head twisting to view the scuffle at the front door. Frau Wendt struggled on the bed, her arms pinned down by one of the men. Her dress had been ripped apart, skin exposed, the savage red imprint of a hand against her breast. The half-naked man above her rolled to one side, his head also turned to the door. Beside the bed, another man waited his turn, laughter frozen on his face.

Out of the corner of his eye, Samuel saw a boot swing at his head. Then the world went black.

Samuel opened his eyes. He could feel a warm trickle of blood running down the side of his face. His hands were twisted behind his back. Above him the half-naked soldier had swung his legs over the side of the bed, a smudge of dirt above the bristle on his cheek. Samuel watched the man button the front flap of his grey infantry breeches. An inch in front of Samuel's face was the muzzle of a rifle. In his mind he saw the Jaeger officer he'd encountered on the road.

'Which of yer was 'sposed to be keepin' watch?' The man on the bed pushed himself upright as he cursed the other deserters in the room.

Next to his head Samuel could see the boots of the man holding the rifle. Including the man standing by the door and the man guarding the children, Samuel counted five.

''ave yer checked outside, yer arschlecker?' The man on the bed clambered to his feet. For the first time, Samuel noted the corporal's lace insignia on the man's tunic. 'Maybe this weed 'as 'is mates waiting outside for their turn.'

Angrily Samuel started to rise. A sharp kick to his thigh confirmed that a man stood behind him.

The corporal walked from the bed, disappearing from Samuel's view as he approached the windows. He heard the rustle of a curtain being moved.

'Looks like 'e's on his own. Must 'ave walked from the village.'

Samuel tried to turn his head, but stopped abruptly at sounds of a struggle coming from the bed.

'Leave 'er yer filthy pig. I told yers I were goin' to 'have first pleasure.' The corporal's voice boomed above Samuel's head. A pair of muddied boots stopped next to his face.

'You're a damn fool,' Samuel hissed through clenched teeth. 'These children are sick with the pox. Didn't you see the sign in the window?'

'Shut your mouth, hosenscheisser.' The corporal's boot clipped Samuel's shoulder, pushing him over onto his side. 'What d'yer mean the pox? What sign?'

Samuel watched the man on the bed swivel his head back to the windows. He deliberately waited before replying. 'We thought one of the children had scarlet fever, now they're quarantined in case it's the pox.'

'What are you, the village doctor?' Again the corporal lashed out with his foot, catching Samuel in the ribs.

'Yes, I'm a doctor,' he gasped, grimacing at the pain in his side. 'But not from the village, from Königslutter.'

'Who gives a scheissen where yer come from? What about the hure on the bed? 'as she got the pox an' all?'

'I don't know. There was an outbreak of smallpox nearby. We have to check all the village folk.'

'Who's we?'

'The doctors from Königslutter.'

The corporal sneered down at Samuel. 'An' you 'spect me t' believe yer.' He turned to his comrades. 'My guess is the weed wants a bit o' what we're 'avin'. Maybe he comes here regular,' the corporal laughed, 'takes 'is fee in kind, so to speak.' At this, the rest of his men shook off their morbid suspicion of Samuel's words and began laughing with their leader. .

'Get some rope. You,' the corporal turned to the man at the door, 'tie 'im up, and gag 'im secure. Put 'im somewhere 'e can watch. See what 'e's missin'.' The corporal sniggered as he threw his rifle to the man standing next to Samuel. 'This time watch the front door careful or I'll ram the end of that up yer arse.'

The door burst open just as the soldier tried to catch the rifle. Heinz barrelled into the room, his shoulder slamming into the soldier by the door, sending him reeling into the soldier still playing a balancing act with the rifle. Both soldiers fell in a tangle of arms and legs, the butt of the rifle bouncing off the ground and smashing into the nose of the guard from the door. Blood streamed from his broken nose, his scream of pain muffled behind his hands.

The corporal pulled a bayonet from a scabbard lying on the bed. Heinz reached out and knocked the corporal's hand away from the blade. With his other hand he grasped the deserter's neck and lifted him off the ground, squeezing with all the force of his arm and hand. Samuel watched the corporal's face turn purple. The man beside the bed pulled a pistol from his belt and swung it up to aim at the two fighting men.

'Heinz, he has a gun!' Samuel screamed as he rolled towards the rifle.

With a grunt, Heinz threw the corporal at his fellow deserter, the man's arms and legs flailing as he flew through the air before crashing into the other man, sending them both tumbling to the floor, the pistol spinning harmlessly away.

'Stop or I will shoot.' The man guarding the children turned his pistol on Heinz.

'I think not,' Samuel's voice sounded strained as he raised the rifle and pointed it with shaking hands at the man in the corner. 'I will not hesitate to pull this trigger if you don't give up your weapon.'

Slowly, Heinz backed away from the bed, careful not to step in Samuel's line of fire. The soldier guarding the children hadn't moved. His pistol now wavered between the big man and where Samuel lay on the floor.

'I will count to five.' Samuel tried to lick his lips, his mouth dry from the tension. 'One ...' Samuel tried to swallow, '... two

... three ...' his voice sounded cracked and nervous, '... four ...' his finger tightened on the trigger.

'Wait! 'ere, 'ave it.' The man turned the pistol in his hand, holding it out to Heinz. 'Don't shoot me.'

Samuel gently took Frau Wendt's hand. 'You may think you can deal with your devils, and perhaps you will, but beware. If you should ever feel the need to chastise your children because you can't understand their behaviour, remember this day and pause. Then, and only then, should you determine the punishment that they may deserve.'

A tear stained the dust in Frau Wendt's cheek. Awkwardly, Samuel placed an arm around the woman's shoulder. 'Because of my writings I suspect you will always be able to find me, and if you should ever feel the need to unburden yourself, please write to me. I promise I will never fail you.'

Heinz sat on the box seat behind the four horses. In the wagon tray the five deserters were firmly tied with lengths of rope and secured to the sides of the wagon.

Frau Wendt wiped her face with the sleeve of her dress. 'I am grateful, sir, for your timely arrival. I fear that five more minutes and both of those animals would have had their way. For now I will trust in my training and in my God, but I am mindful of what you say.' Frau Wendt turned to look at the open door of her lodgings. Tears streamed down her face. 'As if the war has not already taken enough from us without taking the innocence of my children.'

Gently, Samuel offered Frau Wendt his kerchief, which she accepted with a wan smile. 'Is that how you lost your husband, madam?'

Silently Frau Wendt nodded. 'Yes, it was all so unnecessary. He had already done more than enough. I left the convent to return with him to Magdeburg where he was offered a position at the university. He was a truly brilliant surgeon. Some years later Prince Frederick personally asked him to return to the battlefield and become head surgeon. He was killed by a stray artillery shell whilst amputating a soldier's leg.'

'I am truly sorry, Frau Wendt. Will you be all right?'

Again the petite woman nodded. 'Yes, thank you, doctor. It is sad that your latest discovery should be overshadowed by the unfortunate events of today.'

'It is perhaps premature to call it a discovery just yet. That the belladonna has arrested, even prevented, the scarlet fever in your children gives me hope, but I think we will need to test it further before we can relax. I would also ask that for the moment this be kept as our secret.' Samuel raised an eyebrow at the younger woman. 'I fear that my colleagues would dismiss our little discovery out of hand. I intend to treat my patients without telling them what it is that they are taking, knowing that it cannot hurt them, yet hopeful of a cure.'

22

Samuel knocked on the door of his first patient and was met by the child's anxious parents. Calmly and quietly he handed them a small phial containing a clear liquid. He explained that they should give their sick children no more than a drop of the liquid, morning and night, until the symptoms had gone. 'No more than a drop, mind. Do not be tempted to give them any more because it will not work.'

'How strong is this medicine?' the lady of the house asked anxiously.

Samuel shook his head. 'It is perfectly safe,' he reassured her. 'Even if one of the children drank the whole bottle it could not harm them.'

Thirty minutes later he was knocking on the door of his next patient, where he again carefully explained what they must do, again reassuring them that the medicine could not harm their children, stressing that the exact dosage should be given for the remedy to truly work.

For the next two hours Samuel visited each of the five families, patiently advising them of what he wanted them to do, telling each one that he would return the following day at the same time to record any change. Finally he arrived home, exhausted. Johanna and Heinz greeted him in the kitchen, Johanna hugging her husband to her breast in relief, gently touching the small cut where his head had hit the floor at Frau Wendt's house. Tiredly, Samuel smiled at his giant friend, his unspoken thanks acknowledged with a nod.

The next morning three more anxious mothers knocked on Samuel's door. Carefully, Samuel questioned them for the exact symptoms before providing each one with a small phial of clear liquid, with precise instructions on how to treat their children.

That afternoon Samuel said farewell to Heinz and his stepson before starting the exhaustive work of visiting each of his patients. He arrived home late in the evening to find Johanna waiting for him with a warm bowl of soup.

By the fourth day, Samuel's first patients were already reporting that the symptoms had either gone or had eased enough for the children to start being cheeky again. Other families, where the onset had occurred later, were heartened by the news they were hearing all over town.

On the fifth morning, the apothecaries knocked on Samuel's door.

There were three of them.

von Heller was the tallest. He towered over Samuel, his lank grey hair swept in one line across a cadaverous skull. His friend and colleague, Herr Bismarck, made up in girth what von Heller lacked. The vast roundness of the man was topped by a mass of tight brown curls. Herr Reinhardt, the last of the group, had clearly been elected spokesman, his prim hands constantly washing, the thin moustache on his lip twitching in time with his hands.

Samuel waved them to sit down.

'Doctor Hahnemann, there seems little point in wasting time,' Reinhardt said. Samuel's eyes flickered between the moustache and Reinhardt's hands as the man spoke. 'It is now almost a week since we called on you to advise of our intent to take court action if you did not desist from prescribing and dispensing your own medicines.' Reinhardt stopped washing and ran his thumb and forefinger along the thin black line on his top lip. Beside him Bismarck's curls shook in agreement with his colleague's pronouncement, while von Heller remained ramrod straight in his chair, his eyes boring into Samuel.

'We had hoped that you'd have had the courtesy to acknowledge our visit in some way.' Reinhardt drew inspiration from his two colleagues before continuing. 'Instead you clandestinely flouted our wishes and handed out medicines.'

'Is that all?' Samuel asked

'Is that all?' The veins in Reinhardt's neck appeared ready to burst. 'No, it is not all. We intended to issue a warning. Now you leave us with no option but to proceed to the courts.'

'And the nature of that complaint would be?' Samuel asked.

'That you desist forthwith preparing and dispensing medicines, and that if you continue to practice as a doctor, you only ever prescribe medicines made by the apothecaries.' Reinhardt ran his thumb and forefinger across his thin moustache.

'May I ask why you have bowed to the pressure of the doctors?' Samuel's eyes narrowed as he stared back at the three men.

'How dare you …' Bismarck spluttered before Reinhardt and von Heller raised a hand to caution him.

Reinhardt continued. 'You are badly mistaken. There has been no pressure from the doctors for us to do so.'

Samuel raised an eyebrow. 'Then tell me, why is the medicine I am prescribing and dispensing curing my patients of scarlet fever, when the medicines the other doctors are using, which I presume, sir, their patients are purchasing from your pharmacies, is not.'

'This is preposterous.' Bismarck lumbered to his feet, his face the colour of beetroot. 'How dare you insult us. Is it not enough that you break the rules laid down for centuries? It is our sole right to make and dispense medicines; it is our livelihood, yet you thumb your nose at us. To make matters worse, you line your own pockets with money that should be ours.'

Samuel got slowly to his feet. 'On that point I have to correct you, sir. I may be dispensing my own medicines, ones that I can prove work, mind. But I have not made one pfennig from the sale of those medicines. Every single one of my patients has received their medicine free of charge.'

von Heller rose, his thin snake-like body uncoiling to its full six feet. 'This is clearly preposterous, Doctor Hahnemann, your actions are not only illegal but threaten the very foundations of our business. If you cannot see that, then you leave us no choice.' von Heller paused to regard his two colleagues, who were both nodding their heads. 'In the time it takes to convene the court you will be forbidden from dispensing and giving away your own medicines. You may well need to reflect on this, sir, because you will then be forced to seek our cooperation, if you wish to continue practicing as a doctor.'

PART FOUR

LEIPZIG, 1811–1813

23

'Herr Becker, this is the most delightful of surprises.' Samuel clasped his old friend's hand. 'But what brings you to Torgau?'

Councillor Becker took Samuel's hand between both of his own. 'I decided too many years had passed since you told me what was wrong with our world of medicine.' The Councillor's eyes twinkled as he watched the blush creep into Samuel's cheeks.

'Please do not tease me,' Samuel replied. 'All that is hopefully behind me. For a dozen years I have worked diligently to build my practice and enjoy the security of funds to concentrate on my own writings rather than translating the words of others. Have you read the *Organon*?' he asked with a tentative smile.

'Not only have I read it, sir, but I have read all of the other nineteen books and essays that you have written over the past five years,' Becker replied, pleased to see that time had been kind to his friend. He was thinning on top but what remained grew in long curling loops on the sides and back, his face still surprisingly youthful, his back straighter than the last time they had met.

'Yes, yes, they were all very interesting, but what of the *Organon*? What did you think of that?' asked Samuel.

'Well I ...'

'You agree with the rest?' Samuel rushed on before his friend could finish. 'You agree with the rest who chose to either ridicule it or ignore it. One man called me a charlatan. Can you believe that? Another accused me of being a quack. A quack, indeed!'

'Samuel, calm down. Most of the reviews I have read did not tear at your throat. In fact I have been more alarmed at the silence. It is that which made me hesitate.'

Samuel waved Becker to the comfortable easy chair that nestled in the corner of his study. For a moment both men enjoyed the tranquillity of the small garden that gently intruded through the French doors. Finally, Samuel spoke. 'You are right. I think I would have preferred more name calling than to have to endure the deafening silence.'

'It was not quite deafening,' Becker replied. 'I think the reviews were typical of those you have endured in the past, where ignorance and prejudice has blinded the authors. If my reading is correct most of the criticism centred on the size of the dose, which your critics label as too small to be effective.'

'Bah! What would they know? And who was that condescending fool who proffered that there might be some value in homeopathy for certain individual cases.'

Becker shook his head, mildly amused at his friend's eccentricity. 'I don't remember. But I am intrigued at the name, homeopathy.'

'I needed a word that described my theories. "Like treats like" has been expanded. *Similia similibus* has become *similia similibus curentur*, "let likes be treated with likes". The subtlety of the change is important and I tried to capture that thought with the word homeopathy.'

'I'm sorry, my Latin is not as good as it should be.'

'*Homoios* means similar. *Pathos* ...'

'Disease?'

'Correct. Together the two words gave me homeopathy. Unfortunately the new word gives no suggestion of the process of actually curing each disease,' Samuel waved his hand in the air, 'but it lays the foundation. And anyone with half a brain, which clearly these critics don't have, would then be able to draw the right conclusion.' Samuel noted the look of confusion on his friend's face

'Do you recall the introduction to the *Organon*? I wrote that to obtain a quick, easy and lasting cure you must choose, for every attack of illness, a medicine that can produce a similar malady to the one it is to cure. That is the simplicity of *similia similibus curentur* and the power of homeopathy.'

'Perhaps not so simple if your critics get lost on the first page. Pay them no heed, this time you have excelled yourself in your search for the truth.'

'Thank you.' Samuel's gratitude was heartfelt. 'I must admit there have been times when the loneliness of my quest pushed me to the edge.'

'How long did you take to write the *Organon*?' Becker asked.

'Perhaps a year, once my ideas and my theories were clear. But its genesis? Twenty? Thirty? I translated Cullen's *Materia Medica* twenty-one years ago. around the time that I began experimenting with cinchona.' Samuel stood, crossed to his bookshelf and took down a red bound book. Its spine was two inches wide. He flipped through the pages. 'Even a dozen years ago I could not have written this tome.'

'It does not deserve to be called a tome,' Becker interrupted. 'Some medical texts I would call long and ponderous, but this,' Becker pointed at the book in Samuel's hands, 'the *Organon* lives as much through your wit and your passion as for the knowledge it presents. It is a joy for anyone to read.'

Samuel nodded. 'Thank you. Much of what I have written over the past decade I now see as a precursor to this.' Samuel paused to look out into the garden. 'Only when I was satisfied that I could stand up and defend my theories was I confident enough to write this book.'

'The essay you wrote for Hufeland, that was part of this?' Herr Becker asked.

'*Medicine of Experience*? Yes. That was the true precursor to the *Organon*.' Samuel replaced the book. 'All my convictions were truly stated in that book.' He turned to face his friend. 'Of course it remains to be seen whether my fellow physicians are prepared to open their eyes to what I believe is the health-giving truth. But enough of my pathetic ego. What brings you to this over-protected, overblown fortress?'

'You sound somewhat depressed at Napoleon's attempts to build his defensive line,' Becker said in surprise.

'Only because I came to this town for its peace and serenity.' Samuel's eyes were drawn to the garden once again. 'Everything pointed to a peaceful life until our King decided to throw in his lot with Bonaparte. Now we have every town from Hamburg to Dresden fortified against the allies. Have you seen the ramparts he has built to defend the bridge, or the barges loaded with stone that are moored to the banks of the Elbe? Instead of a peaceful town in the heart of Saxony we've become the next stage for Napoleon's ego.' Samuel shook his head, a wry grin on his face. 'You have done it again, my friend. I ask you a question and you sneakily turn it back on myself so that I'm the one who holds the floor. This time I will not be distracted. Why are you in Torgau?'

'Originally I travelled to Dresden where I had been promised an interview with the Emperor himself.'

'With Napoleon?' Samuel's voice rose in astonishment.

Becker smiled. 'Some poor misguided fool told him of the supposed influence of my humble paper. The invitation arrived on my desk three weeks ago.'

'So what did you make of the man?'

'As it turned out I arrived in Dresden to be informed that he had left to visit encampments to the north. We followed him here only to be advised he had travelled on to Wittenburg. I fear that if we do not catch up with him there I will be forced to cut my losses and return home to Gotha.'

Herr Becker stood and crossed to the French doors. 'It would be a pity if you decided to move on, Samuel. This place has obviously been good for you.'

Samuel joined his friend, the pair of them looking out over the garden. 'Yes, it would pain me to sell. I have puzzled over many intricacies whilst wandering this beautiful garden.'

'If you did move, what would you do?' Herr Becker watched his friend's face as he studied his garden.

'For fifty-six years I have acquired a great amount of knowledge. I think it is time I became a teacher, to share my knowledge. I have written to an old friend at the university in Göttingen. If he can't help I will approach the other universities, or perhaps even start my own college. Rest assured, my friend, you will be the first to know if I move and where I am.'

24

December 3, 1811

Dearest Friend, Councillor Becker,

I believe that you do not know that I am six miles nearer to you. I was threatened to be swallowed up amidst the gigantic ramparts of Torgau and I escaped here to Leipzig. But I do regret the pretty house I have left and the garden around it, where I think I have puzzled out many things for the good of man.

We have settled into a comfortable house in the distinguished Burgstrasse called Die Goldene Fahne. The Golden Flag seems an apt name for my plans to set up an Institute for the Postgraduate Study of Homeopathy. If you would be so kind, I have enclosed an announcement for publication in Der Reichanzeiger. Please

>   send your account of expenses
>   to my new address.
>
>   With Kindest Regards
>   Sam. Hahnemann

Samuel stared at the date at the top of the page. Could it really be forty-one years since he first came to Leipzig, despatched by his father at fifteen to work in a grocery store. He cringed as the memory flooded back. So much had happened since then, he thought, so much.

25

January 25, 1812

My Dearest Friend, Councillor Becker,

Not a single doctor has applied to join my college. I am dismayed that the world has still not awakened to the truth, but I am not bowed. I intend to apply to the Dean of the Faculty of Medicine at the University of Leipzig for permission to present medical lectures. I am convinced more than ever that I must try to persuade the medical fraternity to accept my ways. Perhaps it is through the innocence of youth that this will be achieved, for it is only the heads of the young that are not filled to overflowing with a flood of dogma, and whose arteries are not full of the sludge of medical prejudice.

I hope this letter finds you well.

With Kindest regards
Samuel

Samuel laid down his quill, carefully folded the sheet of paper and placed it inside an envelope before dropping it on top of another, already addressed. He would post the letter to Herr Becker on his daily walk. Perhaps he would even stroll past the university and deliver the other in person.

26

February 10, 1812

Dear Doctor Hahnemann,

Thank you for your letter of enquiry. We note with interest your application for permission to give medical lectures at the university. Unfortunately an external doctor, no matter how well qualified to practice, is not permitted to deliver lectures until he has defended his own dissertation from the Upper Chair. If you wish to take up such an opportunity we will require a surety of fifty talers to be deposited with the faculty. If you were successful in presenting your case you would become perfectly legitimatised and be entitled to advertise your lectures in the syllabus and by way of public announcements.

Once we have received the said funds we will advise you further of the procedures.

Yours Faithfully
Professor Rösenmuller
Dean of the Faculty of Medicine

Samuel read the letter for a second time and then rubbed his hands together. No-one, he vowed, no-one, either before me or after me, will set this place on its heels as I propose to do. And, he promised himself, he would do it without one whiff of controversy.

27

Samuel made his way from the side door. The auditorium was filled to capacity, forcing the crowd to spill into the aisles. A murmur of antcipation rose from the audience as all eyes in the room locked on him. He risked a glance, straining to pick out a friendly face. In the front row Samuel recognised several members of the faculty. A vacant seat waited at the end of the row next to the centre aisle.

To Samuel's right the symbolic Upper Chair towered over the proceedings. Intricate carvings imprinted their shape on his mind, the warmth of the timber flowing onto the panelled walls. Briefly he lifted his head, his eyes taking in the majesty of the glass roof that added to the kaleidoscope of shapes and colours.

Pride swelled in his heart at the sight of Friedrich, who had willingly agreed to act as respondent. Beside his son, Samuel recognised Professor Ludwig, the newly elected Dean. In front of them stood the lectern, the eighty-six pages of Samuel's dissertation already laid out upon it.

A smattering of applause broke out as Samuel climbed the few steps to the podium, but it died just as quickly as the Dean stepped forward to address the audience. He nodded at Samuel and then in a perfunctory manner began his introduction.

'Gentlemen, distinguished guests, fellow members of the faculty, we are here today to witness the dissertation entitled "An

Historic-medicinal essay on treatment and cure with Hellebore of the Ancients". The dissertation will be defended by the author Samuel Hahnemann, doctor of medicine and surgery, honorary member of the Society of Applied Sciences of Mayence, member of the Physical and Medical Society of Erlangan and member of the Royal Economic Society, which flourishes in Leipzig. It will be answered by his son, Friedrich Hahnemann, Master of Arts and Bachelor of Medicine.' The Dean looked up from the paper in his hands. 'Gentlemen, please welcome our guests.'

The Dean shook hands with Samuel as applause rippled through the large auditorium. With a nod to Friedrich, Samuel moved forward and placed both hands on the lectern. He looked down at the first page of his essay before lifting his eyes to peer at his audience.

'I would like to offer my thanks and appreciation to the Dean and the members of his faculty for affording me this privilege.' Samuel bowed to the Dean, who had taken the vacant seat in the front row, and then looked to the back of the large Audience Hall. The number of students and guests, unable to find seats stunned him. His heart soared as he returned his attention to his paper. He turned the first sheet, using the time to calm the beating in his chest.

'The subject of my thesis, to which Dean Ludwig has alluded, is white hellebore. Specifically, I intend to demonstrate not only the efficacy of hellebore, but that it is the same as the much praised and used veratrum album.'

A murmur rose from the audience. The learned scientists crammed into the first two rows passed non-committal glances amongst each other.

'The complete title of my dissertation is given in the Latin, as is the custom. I also propose to present my case in the original and will be supporting my argument with passages from many learned writers over the ages. In each case I will quote in the language of the author to ensure the accuracy of my argument and will then offer my point of contention, or my extension of their commentary.' Samuel paused and adjusted the spectacles on his nose.

'The full title of my thesis is correctly *Dissertatio historico-medica de Helleborismo veterum Quam Gratiosi medicorum ordinis auctoritate in auditorio maiori D. XXVI Junii MDCCCXII defendet auctor Samuel Hahnemann Medicinæ et chirurgiæ Doctor acad. Moguntinæ scientiar utilium societatis phys. Med. Erlang. Et societ. Regiæ œconum. quæ Lipsiæ floret sodalis honorarius Respondente Frederico Hahnemann filio art. Lib. Mag. Etc. med. Bacc.*

Without pause Samuel continued in fluent Latin.

'Hellebore is often referred to as a remedy for insanity and as an emetic, even the term "helleborosus" describes someone who is not in his right mind and who requires quantities of hellebore to sustain any vestige of normality.'

A pin could have been heard dropping to the floor, each man in the room, young or old knew intimately the predilections of the polemical Samuel Hahnemann. Each one waited with a growing sense of anticipation for him to break from his litany of precedent and utter his first contentious words.

Meanwhile Samuel had moved on and was outlining the use of hellebore as a medicine from its earliest traces dating back to 1500 BC. As he followed the transcript of his essay the pages turned into a blur of testimony from the ancient writers. Without breaking from the flow of his text or his argument Samuel quoted Avicenna in the original Arabic. He delivered verbatim, commentary from Galen, Pliny, Oribasius, Herodotus and Ctesias the Coan, Theophrastus the Eresian and many more of the most famous and notable medical writers throughout history. He turned from Greek to German to French, then from English to Italian and then back to Arabic, each recitation dependent on the language of the text he was quoting. With unbridled passion he examined the medical writers in their turn, presenting their views and their knowledge on his subject.

'For centuries,' Samuel continued, 'white hellebore proved to be an incomparable drug capable of producing the most poisonous effects, driving doctors of all ages to exercise the most extreme caution. Yet always in their heart was the hope that through its use they may overcome some of the severest diseases.' Samuel paused for a moment and looked out across the auditorium. Not a single pair of eyes flinched from his, his audience beginning to comprehend the depth of his research and the beautiful simplicity and power of his argument.

After an hour, Samuel's strength was undiminished, his confidence soaring above the rapt attention of his audience. On the pretext of taking a drink of water he looked across at Friedrich, whose proud smile and shining eyes lifted Samuel's heart. He turned back to his task, proceeding to outline how hellebore was first used, to what extent, the time of year and the kinds of diseases for which the ancients used it. He even outlined the types of people it best suited. Meticulously he supported each of his statements, quoting Hippocrates and the famous Æsculapias of antiquity. His sources ranged widely, including naturalists and historians just in case his audience detected a weakness in his defence. Finally he offered his conclusions, quoting from the modern masters themselves, including the revered Haller.

As his last words rang out across the vast auditorium an eerie silence descended on the room. No-one moved. In the entire dissertation Samuel had not once referred to his own principles or beliefs.

Not once had he so much as given the room a whiff of his antagonism towards the practices of his detractors.

The silence stretched until suddenly, a lone pair of hands began to applaud. The sound hung in the air for the briefest second. Then another pair joined in, followed by a third, then a fourth, until the entire room erupted in a cacophony that threatened to shatter the glass roof. Around the auditorium people stood, joining their brethren propped against the walls. The movement spread like a wave until only the faculty members remained seated.

Samuel stared down at the Dean and his colleagues, mesmerised, watching their hands come together in polite applause.

Slowly Professor Ludwig climbed to his feet and turned to his associates, silently gesturing for them to join him. One by one each of them stood, their hands maintaining a soft, steady pattern. Samuel's heart pounded. Finally the Dean left his place and walked forward to join Samuel on the podium. He offered his hand to Samuel, then turned to the audience.

The Dean beckoned for silence and patiently waited, but the applause continued. 'Gentlemen, gentlemen, thank you.' Gradually the applause began to subside until only a smattering continued in the middle of the hall. Then they too quietened. 'Gentlemen, distinguished guests, thank you.' The Dean turned to face Samuel. 'Doctor Hahnemann, I congratulate you on an erudite dissertation, eloquently and intelligently delivered.'

A low murmur rose from the crowd at the inadequacy of the Dean's words. Again the Dean held his hands in the air. 'Please, gentlemen, all of you understand the rules. It is not my place to comment on the worthiness of Doctor Hahnemann's paper until the faculty has conferred. For the moment I feel it appropriate to say that everyone in this room has just heard one of the finest philological dissertations they are ever likely to hear.' A swell of approval coursed through the hall. 'Also, without doubt, the good doctor has provided this school with one of the most accurate historical compilations of medical facts it is ever likely to receive, an occurrence which is very rare indeed. Now, with your indulgence,' Professor Ludwig looked around the room, 'I propose that we retire in order for the faculty to discuss Doctor Hahnemann's credentials as a lecturer.'

One by one the members of the faculty trooped out through the side door leaving the audience bemused, taken aback by the abrupt end to proceedings. Samuel turned to Friedrich, equal parts of bewilderment and satisfaction on his face, the look mirrored by his son. Around them the crowd began to disperse.

A single figure detached himself from the departing audience and made his way forward to the podium.

'Doctor Hahnemann, you may not recall me. We met many years ago in Molschleben. Otto Schaefer.'

Samuel peered down at the portly man standing in front of the podium. 'Herr Schaefer, yes, of course I remember you. We shared some most edifying discussions. You do me a great honour by attending today. In fact I was quite overwhelmed by the numbers.' Samuel waved his hand towards the people in the room. 'However, I suspect that some may be feeling slightly miffed by the reluctance of the faculty to endorse my words as readily as they did.'

Otto Schaefer laughed pleasantly. 'I suspect that no matter what the good Dean had said there would have been some who would still not be happy.' The apothecary looked around the hall nodding at some of the members mingling together to discuss the last two hours. 'Frankly, I must admit to being somewhat surprised myself.'

'Surprised? Surprised by what?' asked Samuel.

Schaefer indicated the auditorium. 'I suspect a great number of your audience came here in the hope that you would live up to your reputation.'

'My reputation?' Samuel bristled, praying his face would not betray the thumping of his heart. 'Hopefully I have proven what I needed to do today, regardless of whatever anyone else may perceive my reputation to be.'

Schaefer smiled indulgently. 'I think you are quite correct when you acknowledge there is room for conjecture.'

'I made no such acknowledgment, Herr Schaefer.' Samuel blustered, anger beginning to take over from his deception.

Schaefer continued as if he had not heard the interruption. 'I suspect half of your audience knows you for your reputation as an outspoken critic of what the faculty stands for.' Schaefer nodded towards the door through which the faculty had disappeared. 'I think they hoped you would add grist to the mill. Others know you for your writings and your capacity to think. Maybe they hoped that you might add to your already burgeoning precepts on homeopathy. There may even have been some in the room who had absolutely no preconceived idea whatsoever about what you would say today.' Schaefer's eyebrows threatened to disappear into his hairline, 'although I doubt it.' The incredulous look on the apothecary's face was replaced by a gentle smile. 'Yet, as you witnessed from the ovation, not one person in the room appears disappointed. As for me, I sincerely pray that the faculty has the wisdom to recognise your capacity to inject new ideas and thought into the university for I have decided to return and spend a further year studying. I would very much look forward to attending the lectures given by Professor Samuel Hahnemann.'

Samuel lowered his head. 'Thank you, Herr Schaefer. My apologies if I appear a trifle sensitive. I am sure you can appreciate the labour that has been required to prepare my dissertation. Like my audience, I had perhaps hoped for a more immediate response from the Dean.'

Three men stood behind Schaefer. The tallest of the three stepped forward, thrusting his hand towards Samuel.

'Doctor Hahnemann,' the newcomer said. 'My name is Kirk. Allow me to congratulate you for the magnificent way in which you handled yourself today. Your wisdom in steering a moderate course has done you great credit. The comments amongst my own group of colleagues attests to that, some of whom are not as liberal or progressive in their thinking as I am.' A smile played at the corners of Kirk's mouth. 'Today's dissertation was — how would the faculty say it? — an interesting contribution to the history of modern science, one diligently collected and critically delivered. I thoroughly enjoyed it. More to the point, I enjoyed watching your tactics in winning over the Dean and his members. I have no doubt that you will be lecturing by Michaelmas. I may even have to take time from my schedule to attend.'

A slight blush came to Samuel's cheeks. Self-consciously he raised his hand to stroke the sides of his face. 'It appears that my tactics may not be quite as subtle as you two gentlemen give me credit.' Samuel looked from Kirk to Schaefer. 'That you have both clearly seen through my intentions causes me to wonder whether the faculty may also consider that possibility when they come to their decision.'

'Oh, I don't think you have any reason to worry about that,' said Kirk. 'Given your reception today the faculty will be hard pressed to find any objections to your medical claims, except perhaps some trivial issues of a philological matter. And where, my good doctor, have you ever met two philologists of the older languages who are ever of the same opinion.'

28

Samuel straightened the white linen scarf at his throat.
His mind drifted back twenty years. He recalled how he'd envied the apothecary's fine Chinese silk scarf that day in the small village of Stotteritz. What was that man's name? Waggoner, Wegner? No, no, Wagner, that was it — Albert Wagner — the same man who had unwittingly delivered the Duke of Gotha's invitation for Samuel to take up the position of asylum manager.

He cleared his throat before turning the key in the lock. Briefly he touched his bald pate; the few hairs that remained had been carefully curled and powdered. His hand moved to his chest, fingering the white linen shirt that matched his scarf. His eyes followed his hand, checking the black waistcoat for any flecks of dirt. A glint from his shining black top shoes caught his eye. Self-consciously he checked that their straps were neatly buttoned to his tailored black trousers.

He pictured the students waiting on the other side of the door, well aware that he was an enigma to some, a figure of amusement to others. The propensity for mirth among young students was as old as time and Samuel was only too aware that his support was more likely to come from these unprejudiced minds than amongst the older doctors who attended his lectures. He had deliberately encouraged their younger minds to embrace his eccentricities knowing that, obtusely, they would also respect his knowledge and wisdom.

With a quiet flourish, Samuel opened the door and took three paces into the room. The lecture theatre was packed, every chair occupied. He advanced another three paces to where a table and chair had been set up. Without a word, he sat and glanced at the book waiting for him on the table. Unhurried, he reached into the pocket of his waistcoat, pulled out his watch and placed it besides the book, each move designed to add wonderfully to the suspense of his performance.

Finally he cleared his throat and looked out across the students. Several of the younger men lifted a hand to hide their smirks, a twinkle in their eye. Samuel smiled at the frowns worn by some of his older audience.

He picked up the *Organon* and cleared his throat.

'The third principle of homeopathy, relates to the prescribing of homeopathic medicines. In traditional medicine the physician prescribes according to the physical symptoms displayed in the patient. In homeopathy the physician prescribes individually by a study of the whole person, according to their basic temperament and responses. The physician must consider not just the physical but also the circumstantial.' Samuel paused, ensuring he had his audience's attention. 'For example, does the patient prefer to be alone or in company? Is the patient artistic or practical? Does the patient prefer hot or cold climes? These and many other pertinent factors are part of a critical examination that demands nothing of the practitioner except freedom from bias and healthy senses.' Samuel added as if in afterthought, 'Oh, and, of course, one needs to be attentive while observing and to exhibit fidelity in recording the image of the disease.'

A titter broke from the back of the room. Samuel relaxed, enjoying the attention of the majority.

'Indulge me,' Samuel continued, 'whilst I read a short passage in which I encourage the physician to allow the patient to talk, even to encourage the patient's family to add their observations.' Samuel opened the book at his mark and began reading.

'The patient complains of the process of his ailments. The

patient's relations tell what he has complained of, his behaviour and what they have perceived about him. The physician sees, hears and notices through the remaining senses what is altered or unusual about the patient. The physician keeps silent, allowing them to say all they have to say without interruption.

'When the narrator has finished what he wanted to say of his own accord, the physician enters a closer examination of each particular symptom by reading through the single symptoms reported to him and asking for particulars about this or that.'

Samuel's eyes embraced the students in the room. 'I am sure you can see the value of such a determination. The physician makes his examination without ever asking a question that could put words into the patient's mouth, or that could be answered with a simple yes or no. In this way we eliminate the potential for the patient to affirm something untrue or even half true, or give them any chance to deny something that really exists out of some mistaken desire to please the physician.'

'Doctor Hahnemann, surely you are not suggesting that our physicians do not undertake the most scrupulous examinations?' The interruption came from the side of the room. A tall, thin man leaned back in his chair, his long legs stretched out before him. Samuel noted with surprise that it was the same man who had introduced himself after his dissertation on hellebore so many months before. Samuel tried to recall the man's name.

'I'm sorry, er, doctor ...'

'Kirk, Joseph Kirk, we spoke briefly after your dissertation.

Samuel nodded. 'Yes, I remember your kind words. My response to your question is very simple. Our current training only requires physicians to deal with the physical symptoms that are presented to them. In turn, the doctor then makes an educated assessment of the symptoms and the likely cause, and prescribes accordingly. What I am explaining is the need to understand more than just the immediate symptoms on display, that the root cause is most probably elsewhere and the physician must dig accordingly.'

'If one accepts that the illness is elsewhere, surely that is the sticking point of your argument.' This time the interruption came from the opposite side of the room.

Samuel turned to face his new protagonist. He recognised the aesthetic looking student from previous lectures who had taken an aggressive objective position, questioning from both sides of the argument at every opportunity. At times Samuel had despaired at the man's attack, at others he'd felt vindicated in his beliefs.

Cautiously he waited to see if the man would add a comment. When none was forthcoming Samuel took a deep breath.

'I am always intrigued when a law student attends a medical lecture. The sharp incision of the legal mind adds a new dimension to that particular expression.'

The youngsters in the audience giggled, several permitting full-throated laughter to ring out. Samuel allowed himself a smile, ensuring it did not become self-indulgent.

'It can only be the sticking point of my argument,' Samuel continued, 'if my fellow physicians agreed with my contention that they must also investigate the whole person. Which, I can assure you, they will not. When confronted by a sudden stomach upset accompanied by constant and repulsive belching, the majority of my colleagues will diagnose some kind of deteriorated stomach content and prescribe a suitable emetic. But, once administered, does the patient instantly respond in a healthy manner, full of life and cheer?' Samuel held out an arm, entreating a response from one of the audience. When none was forthcoming he shook his head theatrically. 'Only in the rarest instances, I can tell you.'

Samuel replaced the book on the table and turned again to his audience, his arms spread wide. 'Or take the attitude of most of my colleagues towards bloodletting as the treatment for haemorrhages.' The smile slipped from Samuel's face, a small bead of sweat formed on his brow.

'At the base of all disease induced haemorrhages there lies a dynamic mistunement, yet the old school deems the cause to be an excess of blood.' Samuel's voice rose. 'They cannot restrain themselves from undertaking bloodletting in order to carry away the supposed malaise.' The bead of sweat started to roll down Samuel's brow, slithering across an eyebrow before slipping down the side of his face. Samuel wiped it away with the back of his hand.

'Then, when the bloodletting doesn't work, they palm it off on the seriousness of the disease.' Samuel placed both hands on his hips. 'In short, these practitioners believe that nothing could have been done to save the patient and that they have done everything possible.'

Samuel's eyes were wide, his words tinged with anger.

Two members of the faculty seated at the back of the room exchanged satisfied smirks as the subject of their common room conjecture fell into his own trap. .

Samuel calmed himself. Slowly he lifted his hands.

Appearing somewhat embarrassed, Samuel sat down. 'I'm sure you all have read about my opposition to bloodletting.' He looked around his audience. 'I cannot seem to discuss it without getting a trifle, how should I put it?' he muttered to himself, 'wound up, eh?'

With an innocent smile he nodded at his fellow lecturers.

The lecture room emptied quickly. The two faculty members had slipped out before the others. A small group of men gathered around Doctor Kirk. Samuel was surprised to see his old acquaintance, Otto Schaefer, who came forward to greet him.

'Herr Schaefer, what a pleasant surprise. Were you hiding at the very back to avoid my tirade?' Samuel said wryly.

'Doctor Hahnemann, a pleasure as always.' Schaefer smiled politely in return. 'I had heard that your lectures could get a trifle warm. But, with respect, I would call that one tepid at best.' Schaefer's smile widened as he shook Samuel's hand.

'Oh, there have been times when it has reached boiling point in here,' Samuel replied with a wink.

'Then I am truly sorry to have missed them.' Otto Schaefer's face clouded. 'Unfortunately a family bereavement caused a change in my plans to resume studying.'

'I am sorry. May I ask whom?' Samuel said.

Schaefer almost whispered his reply. 'My son.'

'My dear sir ...'

Otto Schaefer held up a hand. 'It is some months now.' Schaefer shuffled his feet. 'My son had been studying to assume some of my duties. That is why I decided I could return to study. Unfortunately he wandered too close to our liberator and became a victim of Bonaparte's push across the River Saale.' Schaefer's mouth was stretched in a grim line. 'I'm sorry, Doctor Hahnemann. It is indeed hard to outlive your son.'

Samuel's hand clasped his friend's elbow. 'I have some empathy with you; I lost my second son when he was only a few months old. Although I could not share periods of fellowship with him, I certainly share the emotion of losing a son.'

For a moment the two men stood in the centre of the room. It was Schaefer who broke the brief silence.

'Perhaps you would join me for an ale? I know of a small inn nearby where the landlord keeps his glasses sparkling and the heads lively.'

29

'When did your son die, Otto? It is only six months since Bona-parte tried to revive his fortunes in our wretched land.' Samuel touched his empty glass. The landlord picked up two fresh glasses from behind him.

'He was returning from his studies at Jena University. He and his friends were seeking accommodation near Altenberg.'

'Bonaparte and his rag-taggle army crossed the Saale in late April,' Samuel said absently, 'and reached Dresden by May 8. So your son must have died in the first few days of May?'

Schaefer hung his head. 'The third. You have a good memory, and you are right to scorn, although to describe the army as rag-taggle is being too polite. Napoleon returned to France after the Moscow fiasco with less than thirty thousand of the seven hundred thousand troops mobilised for the Russian campaign. The army he has managed to raise this year is but a shadow of that mighty force.'

Samuel nodded agreement. Like all true Saxons he had closely followed Napoleon's campaigns, particularly so since their Elector, Frederick Augustus III, had thrown his lot in with the Emperor. 'I have mixed emotions about this new alliance, I hope we don't live to regret our lost neutrality, yet everything I read suggests that Napoleon has the measure of the allied forces. I hear that Schwarzenburg has retired to lick his wounds from the drubbing at Dresden.' Samuel suddenly stopped, aware of the distress on his friend's face. 'I'm sorry, my comments about the war are insensitive, given your loss.'

'I must admit the senselessness of his death still causes me grief. My son and his friends were caught up in a stupid, unnecessary set of circumstances that would never have happened had Napoleon's men been better trained.'

'How so?' Samuel asked.

'This army will go down in history as the most ramshackle Napoleon has ever led. It's rank and file comprises mainly young conscripts, many of whom did not even do basic training on how to use their muskets until they had reached their main staging camp here in Saxony. Most of the officers are either old men who should have been left to their dotage, or youngsters still green from playing hide and seek in their parents' parlours. For that, my son paid the ultimate price.'

'I still ...' Samuel began, falling silent at the look of pain that moved like a ghost across his companion's face.

Schaefer took a deep breath. 'Napoleon has found it impossible to replace the cavalry destroyed by the Russians. In light of this lack he chose to engage the allies using his favourite strategy: a fast moving offensive aimed at deciding the campaign in a single stroke.'

Samuel found himself unable to restrain his comment. 'I had no idea that you were such a keen student of war, Otto.'

Schaefer opened his misty eyes. 'The death of a son turns a man's mind in different directions, Samuel, as I'm sure you will attest.'

Samuel nodded in silent agreement.

Schaefer continued. 'Napoleon was so intent on destroying the allies that he drove his army at breakneck speed across the River Saale. When they engaged the enemy, Bonaparte was surprised by an offensive against his right flank. His troops were amateurs, many of them were cut off from the main force. By nightfall there were hundreds of frightened and hungry men wandering the countryside.' Schaefer stared at a point above

Samuel's head, seeing it all in his mind's eye. 'A group of these men happened on the farmhouse where my son had sought accommodation. There were no leaders to instil discipline and when they demanded food, my son and his friends challenged them to leave the owners of the house alone. A fight broke out. Before cooler heads could calm the situation my son had been shot in the gut by a round-ball. It took him two days to die.'

Samuel gently placed a hand on Otto Schaefer's arm.

Fighting off tears, Schaefer surveyed the inn. 'I fear these memories will be particularly difficult for me over the coming weeks.' Samuel's eyes followed his friend's, noting the uniforms sprinkled amongst the customers.

'Regrettably, I think you are right,' Samuel said. 'The Emperor's troops have been pouring into Leipzig for the past month. My wife has told me that some food supplies have become difficult to obtain.'

Schaefer nodded. 'On my way to the university the streets were clogged with cannons and troop transports. It would appear that Napoleon is setting up camp to the south and I think it very unlikely that Leipzig will be spared.'

30

Samuel's arms were laden with papers as he struggled along the narrow street. He took care to avoid the constant stream of people who had chosen the same shortcut through to the distinguished Burgstrasse. His mind was trying to come to terms with the announcement the Dean had just made, the words still rang in his ears.

'Regrettably I have to advise that the university council has decided to defer the winter term. The situation in Leipzig has deteriorated to such an extent that not even the king himself can give us reassurances.'

One of the lecturers shouted from the back of the room. 'Has the engagement been announced or are we all just going to hide in our lodgings, too frightened to confront the allied army?'

Around him a handful of men joined in, their voices raised above the hubbub.

The Dean raised a hand. 'Allow me to finish. There are at least a hundred thousand of the Emperor's men encamped around the city. It is rumoured that another fifty or sixty thousand are only a few day's march away. Twenty thousand of them are our own Saxon brothers. It is irrelevant whether the engagement has been announced or not.' The Dean confronted the man who had interjected. 'And if you please, sir, why should the Generals even consider it necessary to inform an insignificant group such as ours that an engagement is to take place anyway?'

Angrily the Dean shook his head. 'The university is officially closed until further notice. Return to your families and ensure that you have sufficient provisions to last through what I suspect is going to be a particularly bitter and bloody battle.'

'Samuel? I didn't expect you for at least another hour, perhaps two if you were off carousing with your newfound drinking partner,' Johanna said as she opened the front door and greeted her husband.

'Madam, once again your humour is badly timed.' Samuel smiled briefly. He looked into her tired eyes, aware how difficult it was for families to survive with an extra hundred thousand mouths to feed and succour.

Samuel followed his wife into the kitchen, depositing his load of papers on the table. 'The university is to be closed for the duration. There is even talk on the streets of a curfew from dusk to dawn.' Samuel looked around the large kitchen. 'Where are the children?'

'The three youngest are playing in Eleonore's room, and Frederika is studying. She has become fascinated with some of your medical journals. Caroline went to the shops for me and should be home shortly.'

Her words were interrupted by a bang as the front door was flung open. Caroline rushed into the kitchen, a parcel in her arms, her blue eyes sparkling at the sight of her father.

'Papa, what are you doing home?'

'What is wrong with my being home?' Samuel demanded. 'First your mother, now you. You'd think that the pair of you were up to some mischief.'

'Well, it's just ...' Caroline began defensively.

Samuel gathered her in a hug.

'I was only teasing, my sweet,' he said into his daughter's hair. 'My early appearance is due to the closure of the university and not because I suspected you of anything.'

Caroline leaned away from her father, her eyes searching his.

Samuel smiled sadly. 'Unfortunate, but true. Our French visitors are causing more havoc than simply eating every crust of bread in the city.'

Samuel turned to Johanna. 'Have you been able to gather sufficient provisions, Elise? If there is truth in a curfew we will need to seek refuge in our cellar. I fear that Monsieur Bonaparte intends to make Leipzig a battlefield on a monumental scale.'

31

Over the next few days Samuel and his family fell into an uneasy routine.

The streets of the city were choked with soldiers in the familiar red, blue and white, dragging their feet from days of marching and constant battle. Even the horses appeared leg-weary as they hauled artillery carriages and wagons loaded with troops over the cobbles.

Amongst the wagons walked hundreds of refugees, forced to flee from their homes in other parts of Saxony. Occasionally a herd of cattle pushed the weary footsloggers to one side as their desperate owners sought sanctuary for their beasts.

With the streets clogged, the residents of Leipzig cancelled their plans and stayed at home.

Occasionally an ailing refugee, seeing the sign above Samuel's door, would seek medical care. No-one was turned away. Many returned to the street, their purses no lighter, with a promise to return if their condition did not improve.

On the Thursday following the announcement by Dean Ludwig, Samuel opened his surgery for business promptly at nine. In the first hour, he waited patiently for his first patient, reading notes he'd made on a new proving.

A gentle tap on his door startled him from his thoughts.

'Papa, it is nearly midday,' Caroline said quietly, pushing open the door. 'Mama will be calling us shortly for lunch. But before she does there is something I think you should see.'

Samuel pushed his chair back, leaving the book he was reading open on the desk. He crossed to the door. 'What is it ...?'

Without replying, Caroline turned and walked to the front door. Calmly she pulled it open.

For a moment Samuel stood back, the empty street showing through the open doorway.

'The street, it's empty,' he whispered. 'What ...?' Samuel rushed to the doorway and stepped out. The Burgstrasse was empty. Nothing moved, not even a leaf fluttered in the light breeze. Samuel exchanged glances with his daughter, her face mirrored his own expression of surprise and disquiet.

'What does it mean, papa?' Caroline asked anxiously, her voice as quiet as a mouse.

'Unfortunately I think it means the worst, Caroline. I suspect the battle is about to start.'

Samuel rapped on the apothecary's door, the sound echoing in the empty street. The residence was only a few streets from Samuel's home on the Burgstrasse. Silently he prayed that Schaefer would be at home. His knuckles tapped out a tattoo on the thick wood, his impatience transparent in the knocking.

Without warning the door flew open. 'For Heaven's sake, you'll wake the dead ...' Otto Schaefer stood in the doorway. 'Samuel,' he said, the glare in his eyes softening. 'I thought you must have been Napoleon himself looking for drugs for his men.'

'Unfortunately, no. But he is certainly the purpose of my visit.'

'Well, come in, come in. Can't have you standing on the street while hundreds of thousands of men prepare for battle around us.'

Samuel gratefully entered the house, waiting in the hallway as his host quickly looked up and down the empty street.

'This way, Samuel, I was just doing some work in my study. Perhaps I can offer you some tea.'

'No, thank you, Otto, I don't wish to keep you from your work or from your lunch. In fact Johanna will be expecting me to return forthwith to partake of my own. I came to see if you could enlighten me on what is happening. The streets,' Samuel waved an arm vaguely in the direction of the front door, 'the streets are suddenly empty after weeks of being choked with the Emperor's men. Should we be expecting the worst?'

Otto Schaefer invited Samuel to sit in one of two easy chairs arranged at the front of his massive desk. The beautiful rose coloured piece was inlaid with leather, the timber gleaming from polish.

'I fear so. This morning several reliable sources confirmed that Napoleon had arrived in the city. Apparently he has located his quarters just outside the city gates. A somewhat nervous Friedrich is with him.'

'Will there be a battle?' Samuel asked, 'Your knowledge of these matters is infinitely better than mine. What danger should we anticipate?'

'The next few days will be dangerous times for all of us. I have no doubt that the city's fathers will announce a curfew. There will be criers out this afternoon, mark my words.'

Samuel nodded. 'But what of this war?'

'From all reports the allies have been pulling their net closer and closer. Blücher and Bernadotte crossed the Elbe and began their advance on Leipzig from the north with over 140,000 men. From the south Schwarzenberg is bringing another 180,000. They will catch Bonaparte in a pincer if he is not very careful.'

'And us with him.'

'Yes. I suspect that's why the reports suggest that our king is a trifle nervous.'

'A curse on Friedrich for getting us into this mess. If he hadn't changed sides ...' Samuel shook his head. 'What will Napoleon do?'

'Napoleon is very limited in what he can do. If he tries to

throw all his strength at one of them they will simply fall back and leave him exposed and weakened.'

'Which leaves us in the firing line,' Samuel said glumly.

'Not necessarily,' replied his friend. 'Napoleon gains very little by setting his battle inside the city. As long as the residents keep their heads they should be in no real danger, except from perhaps starvation.'

'Which hopefully most have made provision for.'

'Exactly. And if I am as good at this strategy business as you seem to think I am, then I would predict that Napoleon will make his stand to the south and the east. The river and the swamps make it difficult for the allies to attack from the west. But any student of Napoleon will tell you that such an engagement goes against every principle the man stands for. Napoleon has only once before fought whilst surrounded, in Rivoli. Then the lie of the ground worked to his advantage, enabling him to bottle up the Austrian forces in the Adige Gorge.'

'And here?' Samuel asked.

'The terrain is completely different. Here we have a low saucer of ground cut across by several rivers. Unlike Rivoli, his men will be largely untested and his strategic brilliance will be countered by the advantage that Schwarzenberg and the other Generals have.'

'So the three armies will attack him from three different fronts?'

'Four.'

'Four fronts?'

'Four fronts and four armies. Very little has been heard about the Polish army under Bennigsen. I am fairly sure that the Poles are moving in from the east. So, if I'm correct, our glorious Emperor will be attacked from the northeast, the northwest, the south and the east.'

'Won't Napoleon know that? Your own sources appear to know what is going on. What of his own spies?' Samuel asked, his eyes wide.

Schaefer shook his head. 'History shows that he has been

hampered before with poor intelligence.'

'When do you believe this catastrophe will occur?

'I suspect we will be lucky to see the week's end without shots being fired in anger. I hope you have a stout door on that cellar, Samuel. I think that within forty-eight hours the roar of cannons will make sleep impossible. If the circumstances permit, perhaps we could talk again tomorrow evening.'

32

Schaefer led Samuel into his study where two tall pilsener glasses filled to the brim waited on a cloth napkin.

'Nothing says we can't try to relax, Samuel, even if the business we have come to discuss is a sorry mess.'

'The battle doesn't go well?' Samuel asked.

'Well, Samuel, surely that would depend on whose side you are supporting. If I make the presumption that you are a loyal Saxon and on the side of our glorious King and his ally, the Emperor of France,' Herr Schaefer arched an eyebrow, 'then the answer is no, the battle did not go well.'

Samuel offered a tentative smile, expressing amazement at Schaefer's knowledge of the day's events.

'I make it my business, my friend. People still expect me to open my shop and dispense my wares. Everyone talks. I tell you if I had a sideline in ear muffins I would have done a roaring trade today. Someone must have the market covered.' Schaefer's joke died in the gravity of the situation.

Samuel lifted the tall glass of pilsener and took a quiet sip, savouring the light brew.

Schaefer continued. 'The battle began very much as I had predicted. By all reports Napoleon faced some 350,000 allied troops against his own weakened force. Some say his numbers were as low as 150,000, with less than 30,000 cavalry. It would appear that the Emperor once again underestimated the brilliance of Blücher. Either that or Napoleon gambled he would not face a heavy attack from the north and left only a covering force in that sector of his perimeter.'

'I find it hard to believe that Napoleon could be so heavily outnumbered.'

Schaefer agreed. 'Clearly it forced his hand, but he has underestimated Blücher before. Instead of deploying sufficient men to the north with Ney, he concentrated his main force to the south against Schwarzenberg. I even have it on good authority that, during the height of today's battle, Napoleon ordered Ney to send Southam to bolster the numbers against Schwarzenberg, aiding Blücher's cause even further.'

'And how did Napoleon fare against Schwarzenberg?'

'Word is, the day's fighting was particularly brutal, with Napoleon's forces hit hard by the failure of Southam to arrive.' Otto Schaefer forced a grin. 'Apparently Ney had summed up the extent of his own difficulties in the north and before Southam reached Napoleon, had ordered him to forsake his redeployment and return to help.'

'So the extra corps that Napoleon had banked on never arrived?'

Schaefer smiled grimly. 'The farce of it is that Southam appears to have spent the day marching to and fro without firing a single shot in either sector.'

'Did Schwarzenberg prevail in the south?' Samuel asked with a growing sense of unease.

'No. The battle seems to have ended in a stalemate.'

'Leaving Napoleon to fight another day,' Samuel observed.

'Yes, but I'm not sure for how long. You recall that I spoke yesterday of the terrain, that the lie of the ground offered no advantages to our Emperor?'

Samuel nodded. 'You also spoke of the swamps and the river to the west giving him protection from that quarter.'

'That's right and a stalemate is as good as a defeat for

Napoleon. I suspect he gambled everything on achieving a decisive victory today, and didn't get it.'

'I'm lost Otto.'

'I'm not explaining myself very clearly.' Schaefer apologised and tugged at his chin. 'Let me try and explain what I think Bonaparte's tactics were. The swamp and the river were his only line of retreat. If you've ever been down into that area you'll know that there is only one bridge and one road that leads out from it. So why would he choose to fight in such a potential trap?'

Not expecting an answer Schaefer paused only long enough to take a sip from his beer.

'My guess is that Napoleon realised he was vulnerable and that the only advantage to be served by his inferiority in numbers was as bait.'

'Bait?'

'To draw the enemy into one final and decisive battle. Although he has had his share of victories in this campaign, they have been punishing victories.' Otto looked pointedly at Samuel. 'With his usual arrogance he would have backed his own genius over that of the allies.'

'So that is the end of it?'

'No-one would ever underestimate Napoleon. Even this afternoon there are reports that he has asked his enemies for an armistice to discuss peace terms. Somehow I think his enemies will be too wise for that old ruse.'

'Otto, you never cease to amaze me with your knowledge of these things. Whatever do you mean by "that old ruse"?'

'Only that he has used it many times before. This time I suspect his enemies know exactly where they have him, and they will squeeze until he cries out for mercy.'

'And do you think the mighty Napoleon will do that?'

Schaefer smiled as he reached for his glass.

33

The following morning an eerie silence hung like a shroud over the city. Samuel and his family had slept fitfully during the night, woken on several occasions by the roar of cannons. As soon as he considered it safe, Samuel shepherded Johanna and his daughters up from the cellar into the kitchen where the air was overladen with the stink of gunpowder and mud.

Samuel looked out through the window and watched the rain fall on his beloved garden. Small pools formed in tiny depressions in the ground. Overhead a solid sheet of grey cloud warned that there was little likelihood of a break soon. Yet, even damp and sodden, the garden offered a sense of peace and tranquillity that belied the horror and brutality of yesterday's battle. How long, he wondered, would it take the allies to bring it to an end?

The rain continued to pour as the Lord's day of rest stretched towards midday. Samuel found it impossible to concentrate and by late morning had had enough of being cooped up. The silence in the house matched the silence outside, the lack of noise bringing with it an irrational anger that made Samuel clench his hands in frustration and his heart to beat at a quickened pace.

As soon as this battle is over, he promised himself, just as soon as the last rifle has been fired, I will offer my assistance. Then there will be much doctoring to be done.

A loud knocking at the door interrupted Samuel's thoughts. Turning quickly, Samuel grunted in pain as his knee crashed into the side of the desk. Cursing and grimacing, he limped to the door and pulled it open.

Otto Schaefer stood on the doorstep. Behind him waited a carriage, it's polished timber gleaming in the rain. Samuel recognised the driver as the same who made deliveries for the apothecary. Stoically, the man sat in silence as the rain crashed into the glistening oilskins draped across his shoulders. Still grasping his knee, Samuel smiled sheepishly at the startled look on Schaefer's face.

'Otto, what a pleasure,' Samuel gasped through clenched teeth. 'I banged my knee when you knocked. I'm afraid you gave me a fright.' Samuel's words trailed away in embarrassment.

'Sorry.' Schaefer brushed aside Samuel's greeting, hardly glancing at the offending knee. 'I have come to ask a favour of you.'

'If I can be of help, you only need to ask. Please come inside out of the rain.'

Schaefer pushed past Samuel into the hallway. 'Well, strictly, it's not for me but for the medical faculty at the university.'

'If the faculty needs me for something why wouldn't the Dean approach me himself?' Samuel asked, surprise in his voice.

'I'm not sure this is entirely the doing of the Dean, Samuel. Apparently a Doctor Griesslich has been given the unenviable task of organising the university's church into a military hospital.'

Samuel muttered under his breath. 'You did say, Griesslich?'

'Yes, is that a problem? Apparently the rumours suggest twenty thousand men lost their lives yesterday, with the same number of poor souls wounded.'

'Oh my God!'

'It's devastating.' Schaefer breathed. 'The military hospitals set up in the outlying areas have already been overwhelmed. The university has asked the faculty to gather a team to attend to the thousands of wounded who are pouring in through the city gates. I fear that when the fighting resumes the allies will push the French closer and closer to the city's walls. Whether we are completely overrun depends on what Napoleon does in the next twenty-four hours. Meanwhile, the number of dead mounts as the wounded succumb to their injuries.'

'And they might just as well continue to mount with Griesslich in charge,' Samuel muttered.

'What do you have against Griesslich?'

Samuel ignored the question. 'Tell me. What did you mean when you said that you'd come here on behalf of the faculty? You said something about this not being entirely the Dean's doing.' Samuel scratched his head. 'Surely the Dean would have provided Griesslich with a list of the doctors on his lecturing team?'

Schaefer nodded, an embarrassed look on his face. 'Yes, he did, I saw the list a few hours ago,'

'Was my name on that list?'

Schaefer nodded. 'Yes, your name was most definitely on the list,' and then he added bluntly, 'but for some reason it had been crossed off.'

'Crossed off? What do you mean, crossed off?'

'Well, crossed off. A line had been drawn through it,' Schaefer said with a touch of frustration. 'I challenged Griesslich. I told him you were one of the finest doctors on that list.'

Slowly Samuel nodded. 'Now I understand what you meant when you said it wasn't entirely of the Dean's doing.'

Schaefer lowered his eyes, avoiding Samuel's angry gaze.

'Griesslich and his cronies would have taken great delight in crossing my name off the list,' Samuel said, willing Schaefer to look up. 'They are all allopathic practitioners. Not one of them has any time for me or my principles.' Samuel slammed a fist into the palm of his other hand.

'Samuel, calm down. Shouting won't resolve the matter.'

'You are right, as usual. But whenever I think I am making some progress my critics rear their dragon-like heads and spit fire at me.' Samuel ran a hand across his brow. 'So, Otto, if Doctor Griesslich and his friends don't want me to contaminate their patients, why are you here?'

'Because, like you, I also got angry and demanded an explanation of the Dean.'

'You did what?'

'There are too many men dying to allow a doctor such as yourself to stand idle. Whether Griesslich and his mob like it or not, I could not stand by without pleading your case. So I went and asked Ludwig who had crossed your name off the list.'

Trying hard to restrain his amusement, Samuel clapped his friend on the back. 'And what was the Dean's reply?'

'He had an apoplectic fit. The veins on his neck stood out, his face suffused with colour and his rate of breathing almost trebled. I tell you, Samuel, it was a terrifying sight,' Schaefer said with a broad grin.

'So, Professor Ludwig agrees with your sentiment, eh, Otto? The wounded and dying are more important than the sensitivities of a few members of the faculty. What does the Dean suggest I do?'

'As far as Griesslich and the other members of the faculty are concerned, you need do nothing. The Dean flew out of his rooms as I was leaving. He intended to have a quiet talk with a few of our friends. As for the wounded? We need to prepare the university church to receive them. A meeting has been called for midday and at this rate we shall be the last to arrive.' Otto Schaefer smiled. 'Given what's happened that may be a good thing. It will allow you to make a grand entrance in front of your detractors.'

'It will take me less than a moment to advise Johanna. Perhaps a grand entrance may be a little petty in the circumstances, but I certainly will not be stopped from making my contribution to ease the suffering of these poor souls.'

34

Throughout Sunday, Napoleon and the allies rested. Rumours abounded that Bonaparte was making preparations for a re- treat, while Schwarzenberg and Blücher waited for Bernadotte and Bennigsen to arrive with a further 100,000 men.

As the lull dragged on into the afternoon, many residents of Leipzig came out onto the streets to mingle with their friends, dismissing the rain as a minor inconvenience compared to the confinement of their homes and cellars.

By nightfall the rain had refused to ease, leaving the city and the surrounding ground soggy and miserable.

The following morning both sides woke to another day of cold mist and lashing rain. But as the day unfolded even the rain failed to dampen the sheer savagery and butchery occurring around the city walls.

Cannons roared and explosions rocked the air. The screams of the wounded blended with the shouts and cries of battle as Schwarzenberg and Blücher pushed Bonaparte relentlessly towards the city. Musket and rifle shot peppered the stone ramparts and the houses of the city. More than 300,000 allied soldiers pressed in on the Emperor's remaining army, relentlessly driving the French soldiers backwards.

As night fell on the third day, the badly savaged French force was encamped with its back to the city wall. Less than 100,000 of Napoleon's original 160,000 men were still standing.

Samuel lowered the bed frame to the floor and straightened his back. His top jacket had been discarded, the sleeves of his shirt were rolled back at the wrist. Slowly he stretched, his hands splayed across the small of his back. The vast chamber of the church rose above him, its empty vault filled with the low moans of the wounded and the soft murmurings of those tending them. Beds were ranged along both walls of the nave with a further twin row placed in the centre of the floor, their steel frames backed head to head. Already two-thirds of the beds were occupied.

'Had enough yet, Samuel?' Otto Schaefer stood at the other end of the bed.

'I must admit that when you asked for my help I assumed it was for my skills as a doctor, not as a labourer.' Samuel spoke grimly, knowing only too well his skills were going to be sorely tested over the coming days.

A deafening crash was followed by another, then another, the roar of cannon closing by the moment, the rolling thunder of explosions threatening to blow the eardrums of everyone gathered in the church. Samuel shouted above the bedlam, his heart thumping in his chest.

'Have they breeched the wall do you think?'

Schaefer shook his head, the roar of cannons fading back into the constant layer of rifle fire. 'No, but the allies are gaining ground. Napoleon promised the king he would not allow the allies to destroy Leipzig. Whether he can keep his promise now remains to be seen.'

There was a sudden flurry at the front of the church. Doctor Griesslich ran towards the wide doors where a group of doctors clustered around a young man, his face blackened by soot and soil.

Samuel and Otto hurried towards the front door, eager for news from the battlefield. Griesslich arrived only seconds ahead of them, his heavy jowls shaking under the steel grey of his eyes. He stared at Samuel and Otto before turning to the crowd, waving his arms, imploring them to allow some air to reach the exhausted messenger.

'The Saxon regiments have turned on Napoleon,' the messenger blurted out to the gasps of the men around him.

'What do you mean, turned?' Griesslich asked, voicing the question on every lip.

A deathly quiet descended inside the church.

'A brigade of Saxon hussars and lancers made as though to charge Bernadotte's Cossacks, then suddenly wheeled and turned their muskets and cannons against the French.

'And what have the French done?' Otto asked, his voice rising above the chorus of gasps.

The messenger turned to his questioner. 'What do you think? They have tried to fill the gap left in their line. And when I left, they were holding their own, even against the renewed spirits of the allied forces.

'Then what of the king?' The shout came from the opposite side of the group. Again the messenger twisted his head.

'All I know is that the king and queen were waiting at their palace here in Leipzig.

'What of the battle?' Griesslich asked, his face drained of colour. 'Will it stay outside the city? Or will we see the streets awash with our own blood?'

'It cannot last much longer; the allied forces are pushing Napoleon harder and harder. The Emperor's officers are talking about retreat.'

'But where will they retreat to?' Samuel blurted out, mindful of Schaefer's prediction of two days before.

'I suspect to the bridge at Lindenau,' the messenger answered, turning to look at Samuel in the gathering quiet.

'Then if it is Lindenau, we can prepare ourselves for the worst.' Every man in the group turned to Schaefer. 'I agree with our friend, Napoleon has only one way to retreat and that is to the west of us, it is the only bridge that can give him escape across the Elster. We must prepare for Napoleon's men to fight hand-to-hand with the allied forces through our beautiful city. It is the only way Bonaparte can get his men out.'

35

'Doctor Hahnemann, please wake up.'
Samuel felt the hand tugging at his sleeve but kept his eyes closed, reluctant to give up the sleep that had claimed him.

'Please, doctor, we need the bed.'

Samuel's eyes flew open, the voice achingly familiar.

'What is happening? What!' He blinked at the woman in front of him, her slight figure covered by a soiled smock. Recognition dawned in the flickering light from the oil lamps. 'Frau Wendt? Is that really you?'

Frau Wendt smiled wearily and held out her hand to Samuel. He took it between both his own. For a moment they stared at each other. Samuel was shocked at the weariness in her pretty eyes, tired lines etched into the corners, the crescent shaped scar on her cheekbone showing white against the streaks of grime.

'Madam, what a pleasure to see you after all these years.' Samuel stopped abruptly. 'For goodness sake, where are my wits? Why are you here?'

'I have been helping the Sisters of St Francis. The pastor told us what had happened here. We came to see if there was anything we could do to help,' Frau Wendt answered quietly.

For the first time, Samuel noticed the nun's habits as they moved amongst the wounded. 'But surely their charity asylum can't spare them?' Samuel asked. 'How many have come to help?'

'Three, plus myself. Several other women have offered their services to the Mother Superior. It was with her blessing that we came to see if we could help.' Frau Wendt wiped the back of her hand across her eyes. 'Word reached us that Napoleon had given the order to begin the retreat at eight this evening. We witnessed the corps under Victor and Augereau, along with the ambulances, enter the town. Lauriston, Macdonald and Poniatowski have taken up positions behind the gates to provide a rearguard. The Mother Superior thought your need would be greater than hers.'

'But why are you with them?'

The slip of a woman stared directly into Samuel's eyes. 'Perhaps you have forgotten that it was the Sisters who nurtured my gifts for helping people. Surely I can offer my services when they need me.'

'Of course,' Samuel blushed, 'perhaps I should have said that I had not expected to find you here in Leipzig. The last time we met you lived some distance away.'

'I have lived here for some years, doctor. I have often seen your name in the journals.'

'Then I'm sad you have not felt that you could call on me, if you knew where I was.'

Frau Wendt looked around her. The church was a seething mass of wounded. Doctors hovered over beds, some of which held two patients. In the sanctuary a rough curtain had been hung to give some seclusion to the surgeons, the ragged drapes of cloth and muslin unable to hold back the stench of blood. Behind the curtain a ragged scream reached a horrifying crescendo and was then suddenly cut off. Frau Wendt spoke quietly, her soft words heard clearly amidst the wretched babble.

'I don't think you understand, Doctor Hahnemann, I live at the convent.'

Samuel considered the lady's dress. 'But clearly you have not resumed their calling. What is it that you do at the convent?'

'Exactly what I came here to do. I help care for the sick. The nuns never turn away anyone in need. I truly believe that I can be of more use there than in the village I left behind.'

'I truly respect your dedication and I am sure your help will be a blessing. I fear the worst if the French decide to punish us for the army's desertion.'

'That is unlikely.'

'You seem very certain of that, madam. Who can tell what punishment Bonaparte may feel appropriate for such disloyalty? He could burn the town to cover his withdrawal.'

Frau Wendt shook her head. 'A number of French officers were evacuated to the convent. They agreed that some of their compatriots were in favour of exactly what you propose, but Napoleon would have none of it. Apparently he met with our King this evening, making plans for him to follow Bonaparte and his army. He would rather do that than lose face for the shameful act of his men.'

'So with the king gone what is to stop Napoleon and his men torching the city?' Samuel asked in exasperation.

Frau Wendt remained calm. 'According to his men, Napoleon has vowed not to allow fighting in the streets. It is rumoured that he even petitioned the allies for an armistice of a few hours to allow his men to withdraw in an orderly fashion.'

Samuel raised an eyebrow at the news. 'And?'

'They refused point blank.'

'And Napoleon still insisted that his men not put up any rearguard fight? '

Frau Wendt ignored the scepticism in Samuel's voice. 'Much of Napoleon's army has already withdrawn and is marching on the Lindenau bridge.'

'Nevertheless these men, and ... children,' a small child lay on a stretcher close by, her leg blown half away. 'That child would be the same age as your youngest.'

Grimly Frau Wendt followed Samuel's gaze, and then turned back to him, a bleak look on her face. 'I think you underestimate the time that has passed since I last saw you, doctor. It is more than a dozen years since I left Königslutter. The twins, are now both sixteen. One of them works as a chambermaid in

Dessau, the boy gained an apprenticeship with the newspaper in Magdeburg.'

Side by side the unlikely pair worked through the night. Sporadic rifle fire punctuated the steady murmur of voices inside the church. From the sound of it, the French were holding the allies west of the university. Samuel was too busy and too tired to give it more than a passing thought. Together he and Frau Wendt had cleaned and dressed a score of injuries, some caused by bayonet, many by shot and ball. Most of the men were too weak from loss of blood to walk from the battlefield and had been brought to the church by their comrades, while others had been deposited by the retreating French flying ambulances.

Tears coursed down Frau Wendt's cheeks as she wiped mud and blood from the chest of a young boy whose legs had been blown from under him by a mortar or cannon shell. Deftly she slipped a hand under the single sheet and found the young boy's wrist. Without a word she closed the boy's eyes and turned away from the bed. Samuel signalled for two men to remove the body. He crossed to the tiny nurse and laid a hand on her shoulder. She stood quietly for a moment and then gently touched his hand before turning to the next bed, where an amputee had been returned from the surgeons. Quickly she checked his dressing and then moved onto the next man.

'Do you know the story of Baron Dominique-Jean Larrey?' Frau Wendt asked as the two bent over a man whose arm hung from his shoulder by a thread of skin. Gently she cleaned the man's torso, preparing him for the surgeon. Samuel had already cleaned a second gash in the man's chest, clearing out grit that had become embedded.

'The name is familiar.'

'Larrey was the Emperor's surgeon who developed the flying ambulances. You would find much to admire about Doctor Larrey. Like you, he is a devotee and advocate of good hygiene as an essential part of good doctoring and healthy living.'

'A very wise man indeed.'

Frau Wendt smiled. 'Larrey became distressed at the time it took for the military hospitals to reach the wounded. Usually dying men were left where they fell or at a convenient landmark to be collected after the engagement.'

Samuel replied without looking up, 'I understand the progress of the military hospital could be so impeded by the detritus of battle that often it would take up to 36 hours for the wounded to be tended. By which time many had expired.'

'That is what got Larrey thinking,' Frau Wendt said. 'He saw that the artillery could be mobilised quickly and escape from the clutches of the enemy in the blink of an eye.'

'Perhaps something to do with our warped sense of priority?' Samuel looked up at the woman who worked beside him. She was wrapping a bandage around the eyes of a soldier lying prone on the next bed. He returned his attention to his own patient where he drew scraps of iron from a deep wound in the thigh.

'Quite,' she said dryly. 'Anyway, Larrey approached the Field Generals with the idea of a medical team that could follow the advance guard in the same way as the flying artillery. He proposed that a special carriage be built to be drawn by a team of fast horses.'

'Fascinating, Frau Wendt, but the point of your story eludes me.'

'Have you looked at the cause of the majority of wounds we are required to treat?'

'Of course.' His words were short. Samuel rubbed his forehead tiredly. 'I'm sorry, Frau Wendt.'

The weary woman looked up, a sad smile on her lips. 'There is no need to apologise, everyone is tired and in a state of shock from these past few days.'

Samuel pursed his lips. 'I have noticed there are only a few wounds that have been caused by a blade or a bayonet.' He concentrated his mind, looking for the purpose of Frau Wendt's question. 'Most have been caused by ball or shot. In fact now that you mention it, most have required amputation.'

Frau Wendt nodded. 'Men impaled by a bayonet are unlikely to make it from the battlefield. Those with flesh wounds from the same weapon can often treat themselves, or at least make their own way to the hospital. Before the flying ambulances, most of the wounded you see on these tables would not have made it from the battlefield. They would have died waiting for the military hospital to reach them, died from loss of blood or shock, or a combination of both. Now these men have a chance to live, even though many of them might not thank us for the life they will return to.'

'You are a remarkable woman, Frau Wendt. At my age there are not many who can give me such a timely lesson in medicine.'

Shortly before midday Samuel was again woken rudely from a nap. His head had rested on the pillow for less than an hour when a mighty explosion rocked the city. The windows of the church rattled, men and women dived for the floor. Others remained standing, too shocked to move.

Having ordered his army's retreat, Napoleon had left his quarters and ridden to the last bridge, known as the Millbridge. There, he dismounted and ordered that a charge be laid under the bridge and that it be blown once the rearguard had passed. He then sent orders to Macdonald and Poniatowski to hold the city for a further twenty-four hours to allow the main body of men time to get across the bridge. Satisfied that his orders had been carried out, Napoleon remounted. He had gone barely a thousand yards before a mighty explosion nearly knocked him from his mount.

Whether the sapper had misunderstood his instructions, been panicked or was part of more sinister mischief could not be determined. But the bridge had been blown, leaving 20,000 men and more than 200 artillery pieces to the mercy of the closing allies.

Samuel lifted his watch from the fob pocket in his waistcoat. Through drooping eyelids he was surprised to see that it was already past six in the evening.

The street outside his home was littered with debris. A broken wheel lay across his doorstep, the wagon it had deserted lay broken, twenty yards away. Tied bundles of baggage spilled over the tilted wreckage. Surprisingly there were no bodies amongst the litter.

Word of the savage fighting that had see-sawed through Leipzig had filtered through to the hospital. The French had fought valiantly to halt the allied push, defending every street corner as if it were their beloved Paris. The last of the casualties brought to the university church had told of the debacle as French soldiers reached the final line only to find their escape route blown. As Samuel swabbed the hole in one man's chest, the soldier screamed and babbled about how he had seen Marshall Poniatowski, in a desperate attempt to avoid the slashing blades and lances of the pressing allied cavalry, ride his wild eyed steed into the murky waters of the Elster. The man fainted before Samuel could learn whether the gallant Pole had survived his leap.

He swiped the back of his hand across his eyes, taking a deep breath, which became a wide yawn. Wearily Samuel dragged himself up the steps of his house. As he was about to open the door a wave of sound pushed up the Burgstrasse. The thunder of horses was joined by the blare of trumpets. Advancing at a smart clip rode a group of officers at the head of a troop of cavalry and cuirassiers, their gleaming helmets topped by flashes of red and green. At the front of the group a tall man stood in his stirrups, his cocked tricorn hat topped by a plume of black and yellow feathers. Immediately behind him rode a flag bearer, his flag and attendant pennants announcing the arrival of the Austrian Field Marshall, Prince Karl Phillip of Schwarzenberg. The mighty General's weary eyes swept across the growing crowd and locked onto Samuel's. Smartly, the Austrian brought his hand to the forepeak of his dress hat and briefly saluted.

36

'I have had enough, Otto. This latest insult is the last of it. The fools in the faculty can fight this battle on their own.'

'Calm down, Samuel, please.' Schaefer pleaded with his good friend. The two men were seated in Schaefer's study. A week had passed since the victorious allies had pushed Napoleon across the Elster and, from all reports, out of Saxony for good. People were already celebrating Napoleon's retreat, believing the battle at Leipzig was the final and decisive nail.

'At a time when I should be able to enjoy peace in my beloved Saxony', Samuel continued, his friend's plea going unheeded, 'perhaps peace for the first time in my life. Even this I cannot enjoy because another peril confronts us. And now you tell me that my colleagues are standing against my rights to treat these poor folk.'

'Calm down. You are rambling in your anger.'

'How would you react?' Samuel seethed. 'I warned them. Even as the last of Napoleon's army was fleeing through the marshes of Lindenau, I told them that we had not seen the end of it, that typhus would follow.'

'And you were right, Samuel. As usual,' Schaefer muttered under his breath, 'but you cannot turn your back on your patients, or the poor souls in the hospitals who are suffering from this accursed plague.'

'It is not a plague, Otto. Please do not call it such or you will panic everyone. It is reaching epidemic proportions, I grant you. But we can treat it, even though these fools are doing everything they can to make it worse.'

'Samuel, please. It is only the same fools who spoke out against you to Griesslich. When I approached the Dean then, he listened. The people who count will listen this time. Trust me. In fact I wonder if it might not be wiser for me to act as mediatory.'

'Tell me why I need a mediator to speak to the Dean?' Samuel stood, almost spilling the glass of pilsener in his hand.

'Because, as usual, my dear friend, you speak with your heart rather than your head. If you are so convinced that you can treat this damned curse homeopathically then you must have the chance. If for no other reason than to silence your detractors!' Otto guided Samuel back into his chair before continuing. 'But you won't get the chance unless you remain calm and coolheaded. For goodness sake, you've shown up these foolish people before. I have every confidence that you will do so again.'

'Please be seated.' The Dean waved a hand at a chair in the middle of his wood panelled reading room. 'It is good of you to come.'

Samuel nodded at Dean Ludwig as he lowered himself into the softly upholstered chair.

'Herr Schaefer has spoken to me about your belief that you can treat typhus homeopathically,' The Dean said.

Samuel nodded, not trusting his tongue.

'As I think you know, Doctor Hahnemann, you have ... a number of critics within the faculty.' The Dean scratched his chin.

Samuel restrained himself, remembering the words of his friend. Wisely he allowed the Dean to struggle with his embarrassment.

'You know as well as I do, Doctor Hahnemann, that not everyone sees things through the same eyes as you.' Ludwig paused, half expecting an explosion from Samuel. When none came, he continued. 'But we are not all of the same cloth, and I certainly am grateful for your fortitude and professional assistance during the recent bloodshed.'

Slightly mollified, Samuel loosened his grip on the Dean's furniture.

'Perhaps, you would be kind enough to enlighten me on what you believe to be the proper treatment and care for typhus?' With the question out in the open the Dean hesitated, wondering if Samuel's silence would continue. Finally Samuel nodded, enabling a relieved Dean Ludwig to retire behind his desk.

'Professor, we both know that typhus follows the trail of war and that there have also been outbreaks of typhoid fever. Much work has been done to prove that there is a difference between the two. I am blessed to be able to read many languages and have seen the work of physicians that may still be unknown to many of our own doctors. There is much conjecture that, whilst both typhoid fever and typhus manifest their symptoms in the same way, they are spread by different means.'

Dean Ludwig nodded. 'Yes, I have seen some of the conjecture. But as I understand it there is nothing absolute. No-one has yet come out and clearly differentiated between them. Whatever you choose to call it, the disease presents itself with a fever, a rash over most of the body and severe headaches.'

Samuel nodded patiently.

'I agree wholeheartedly, Professor Ludwig, but the conjecture suggests that there are two ways, at least, that such disease is spread, and without question they both proliferate from similar unsanitary conditions.'

'So what is your point? How does this change the fact that we are faced with a second major calamity within as many weeks.'

Samuel continued. 'There is common agreement that, whether it be typhus or typhoid fever, hygiene and sanitation are critical to the treatment.'

'I'm not sure I understand, doctor.'

'Last year I read a dissertation in Greek that pointed to the presence of lice on the bodies of typhoid victims. The doctor diagnosed the outbreak as typhoid, with the disease transmitted by polluted drinking water. Yet no-one questioned the presence of the lice and assumed, as we all do, that the infection had been passed by human contact.'

'And your point is? the professor added a trifle irritably.

'I cannot prove it, but I believe there is sense in the conjecture that typhus is passed on by other means, probably louse or fleas or some other parasite.'

'And your proof, doctor?'

'I have none, only my intuition, and of course my absolute belief that most of the ills of the modern world are unambiguously tied to cleanliness as much as Godliness.'

'There is no need to take our Lord's name in vain.'

'You are right. But please, allow me to explain.' Samuel responded, attempting to sound contrite. 'Many years ago, I achieved some minor success in using belladonna to treat an outbreak of scarlet fever.' Dean Ludwig nodded. 'However, I am convinced to this day that a significant part of that success lay in my instructions to keep the patients isolated. In the case of typhus I suggest that isolation is as critical as it was for the treatment of scarlet fever, but I also believe we need to be particularly alert to the personal cleanliness of those infected. It is a key part of the treatment, and necessary to reduce the disease's spread.'

'And pray tell, Doctor Hahnemann, how do you propose to do that? Thanks to Bonaparte our hospitals still overflow with the casualties of that slaughter. We don't have the people to care for the wounded, and now this.'

'Unless we do, Professor Ludwig, I fear that the toll from this typhus outbreak could top the number killed on the battlefield.'

'I think you exaggerate, sir.'

'Exaggerate?' Samuel stood up, finally unable to control his anger. 'The aftermath of the fighting in Dresden four months ago has already left more than fifteen thousand dead from typhus. The doctors there are predicting the toll will exceed twenty thousand. Torgau is the same; tens of thousand's have already died. And those figures are only the civilians; they don't include the number of deaths amongst the military.'

Samuel stood in the centre of the room hands on his hips, momentarily out of breath. Across the desk Professor Ludwig's face had drained of colour. Seeing the look on the Dean's face Samuel calmed himself. 'You were not aware of these figures, sir?'

'I ... I have been occupied.' The Dean shook his head. 'I'm sorry, that is very lame, but things have not been the easiest here in Leipzig, as you well know.'

A stab of guilt hit Samuel, aware that the Dean had worked virtually non-stop since the battle. 'No, it is I who should apologise, Professor Ludwig. The figures have come through my good friend Herr Schaefer's network.' Samuel smiled awkwardly. 'I have my differences with the apothecaries, as most would attest, but I must admit admiration for their communications.'

Professor Ludwig stood up behind his desk. 'Doctor, regardless of what some on the faculty may say, you have my full support. Your assistance in dealing with this ... this outbreak will be gratefully appreciated by the city, I am sure.' The Dean sighed deeply. 'Unfortunately I cannot guarantee that your plea for improved attitudes towards hygiene will be heeded, but I certainly will not stand in your way of treating your patients homeopathically.'

37

'Frau Wendt, please, we will need more water. Each of these men must be washed from head to toe. And the beds need to be stripped, and the sheets and blankets laundered ... tell the orderlies. They must make sure that all the lice are cleaned from the patient's skin.' Samuel bent over a young soldier whose face was flushed red. Sores had already erupted on the man's cheek

'Doctor Hahnemann, I have just finished explaining. This is a convent, there are no orderlies, only myself and one novice — and yourself!' Frau Wendt replied, her voice catching in her throat as she surveyed the thirty beds in the room, each one occupied by a stricken man or boy.

'What do you mean, no orderlies? How else can we expect to get all these men washed down?' Samuel stormed. He calmed himself and continued his instructions, appearing to pay no heed to Frau Wendt's chilling reminder. 'We must also remove their clothes,' he continued as if chanting catechisms, '... have them burnt. The clothes and the bed linen are our worst enemy. We must wash the linen in boiling water. The clothes must be incinerated.'

'Doctor, calm yourself.' Frau Wendt gently took his elbow. 'All you are doing is upsetting the patients.'

Slowly Samuel took control of his ragged breathing. 'As always you come to my rescue, madam. You are right, but there is no time to waste. These men are poisoning themselves whilst we stand here and talk. Lice and fleas, not polluted water, is the cause of this. 'These lice have swarmed everywhere Napoleon has waged his wars. The rats and the mice feast on the waste of human garbage. Then the parasites leave their filthy hosts and begin to feed on the men themselves. After the lice have bitten, the patient scratches, breaking the skin and probably spreading whatever poison is in the bite. Or perhaps it is just the faeces of the damn things that harbours the sickness.'

'I think I understand but without sufficient help it will take me hours to wash this many men, never mind changing the bed linen as well,' Frau Wendt replied, her nose wrinkling at the sour smell in the air.

'Of course I will help ... Where is the nun?' Samuel demanded, his anger beginning to boil over again.

'Please, Samuel,' Frau Wendt whispered, 'please, the patients.' Gently she pulled him away from the bed. 'I asked her to bring fresh water, and ... emetics to purge these men.'

'What!' Samuel shouted, his face as red as some of the patients. Samuel waved his arm towards the door at the end of the room. 'I forbid her from bringing any such medicines into this ward. Please find her, Frau Wendt, tell her to bring Bryonia and Rhus Tox. And hot water and soap. And hurry!'

Frau Wendt found the nun in the convent dispensary, her arms filled with bottles and equipment. Abruptly she turned the young girl around and started unloading the paraphernalia back onto the bench, urgently whispering Samuel's instructions. An elderly nun watched silently. Frau Wendt turned to her and explained what she required. Without a word the nun beckoned Frau Wendt to follow her into the herb garden.

On her return, Samuel had already stripped half the men of their clothes, the offending articles thrown onto a pile in the corner.

'Take those and have them burnt,' he instructed the harried young novice. 'Use a sheet to bundle them in. Then come back for the rest.' He dismissed the young girl. 'Frau Wendt, can you please help me finish undressing these men. Every shred of clothing must be removed. Then the linen. Then finally we must wash down every surface to make sure none of these men can be re-infected. I don't intend to allow even one of these men or boys to die. Not one, do you understand me?'

Samuel pushed himself up from the bed. Carefully he stretched his back, the muscles refusing to straighten. The final dose had been administered nearly fifteen hours after he had walked into the small room. Around him lay twenty-three men and seven young boys. The men ranged in age up to fifty, a rag-tag mix of Saxon soldiers and citizens. The young boys were aged between eleven and fourteen, all of them brought in from the streets where they had been earning a measly few pfennigs from the town's councillors to return order to the city. He felt a gentle tug at his sleeve. Frau Wendt stood beside him, behind her he could see the young novice. The exhausted girl had fallen asleep sitting upright in the hard-backed chair at the head of the room. A pail of water stood to one side of her, a mop propped up against it.

'Samuel, you must get some rest. It's now two in the morning. You look exhausted.'

'No more so than you, my dear lady.' Samuel tried to smile. 'But there is still work to be done. With only three of us we must make up some kind of roster to remain vigilant. At least until I can persuade the Dean or the Mother Superior to give us more hands.'

'I don't think you will have much success in persuading the Mother Superior to give you assistance. She is already struggling to meet the demands on our small asylum. There are still a great number of wounded here.' Frau Wendt spoke quietly, her eyes taking in the patients in the ward, constantly looking for anything untoward.

'Do you know, Frau Wendt, after all these years I have never heard your first name. It gives me great pleasure that you have finally chosen to call me Samuel. But, I cannot reciprocate.'

Samuel's smile was gentle, his eyes drooped with fatigue.

'Christina. My parents christened me Christina Henrietta,' she said tenderly. 'I seem to recall that your eldest daughter was also named Henrietta.'

Samuel nodded. 'Your memory, like everything else, does you great credit. Christina. It is a beautiful name, and well worthy of such a beautiful person.'

'You'll make me blush, as tired as I am. Enough of this sentimental time-wasting,' Christina Wendt admonished him, the soft smile on her lips becoming wider. 'You are right. We do need a roster, and your name will not be on it.'

'Don't be absurd, Christina. I am adamant that I will do my share.'

'Your share, I suspect, will be greater than all of ours combined if the numbers keep mounting. Not only will you have the task of directing treatment here, but I suspect you will also find yourself attending to many victims in their own homes.' Christina laughed softly. 'I would also be surprised if there is enough bryonia in all of Leipzig to satisfy your need, so that will be another task for your persuasive tongue.'

'Oh, I think I know someone who will be far better equipped than I in that department. Herr Schaefer owes me a favour after getting me involved in all of this in the first place.'

Samuel smiled and then became serious once more after noticing Christina scratch absently at her side. 'We have been exposed to the same parasite that has afflicted these men. It is absolutely essential that we are scrupulously clean at all times. The clothes we are wearing must be washed in boiling water, and washed again after we come into contact with any new patients.'

'And how long will we need to maintain such a strict regimen?'

'I truly don't know, Christina. The eruptions we see on the bodies of some of these men and children occur after three or four days. Most will have extremely dangerous fevers for 12 days, then it will fall very rapidly. Up to half of them usually die.'

Christina Wendt narrowed her eyes. She nodded. 'That is

what I have heard. I did not want to dampen your confidence earlier when you vowed not to lose any of these patients.' She lowered her voice. 'We are going to lose a large number, Samuel, no matter how diligent we are.'

Samuel took Christina's hands in his own. 'You are the last I would have expected to hear speak such words. Have you already forgotten how we treated your children when they were touched by scarlet fever? And that it worked. Why do you forsake me now when I need your confidence more than at any other time?'

Tears flooded Christina's eyes and cascaded down her cheeks. 'I do not forsake you, Samuel, I trust you. But there has been so much death. Thousands of people have died from this disease. How can one doctor and two novices make any difference?'

'We will make a difference, Christina, if my theory is proven right.'

PART FIVE

LEIPZIG, 1816 – 1817

38

'Otto, come in, come in.' Samuel grasped his friend's hand in both of his own and hauled him in from the doorstep. 'It's been too long. What is it? Three, four years? I'm so glad you could take time from your busy schedule to join our little dinner party.'

'I could never be too busy to catch up with good friends,' Otto Schaefer said warmly. 'And I see you are still prone to unashamed exaggeration. It is perhaps a little over two years. I left Leipzig for Dresden not long after the battle.'

'It seems much longer.'

'It was not that long after you received accolades from the city's fathers for your work with the typhus victims.'

Samuel's laughter sounded a little strained. 'Perhaps one of these days the medical fraternity will have the same wisdom as the councillors and not ignore the fact that we lost only two of nearly two hundred patients. And one of them an elderly man already frail from the ravages of time.'

'Come, Samuel, even in Dresden several doctors I know were applauding your success. Anyway, stop putting so much store in the opinions of your colleagues and start worrying about what your patients think.'

'It is good to see you, Otto. Please come in and meet my

guests. I think you will find them a little more supportive of my, er, idiosyncrasies than my medical colleagues.'

Schaefer followed his friend down the passage. He could hear the murmur of voices in the sitting room. 'It sounds like the party is off to a merry start.'

Samuel glanced over his shoulder. 'I should warn you that we will be the oldest amongst those gathered here this evening and I can certainly promise you will not be bored witless by a bunch of narrow-minded homeopaths.'

'Those that I know have never struck me as being narrow-minded,' Otto responded.

Samuel paused at the entrance to the room, a twinkle in his eye. 'And how many homeopaths do you actually know, Otto? One?'

There were eight people in the drawing room, most of them in their early twenties. One young man, talking to Johanna Hahnemann, could not have been more than twenty. Beside him sat a young lady, who Otto recognised as Samuel's daughter, Frederika. 'Come in and meet my fellow missionaries, Otto,' Samuel whispered, his eyebrow raised above a broad grin.

Otto bowed. 'Madam, it is a great pleasure to see you again. I must congratulate you on how content your husband appears.'

Johanna kissed Otto Schaefer on the cheek. 'I don't think I can take all the credit for his disposition, Herr Schaefer. For a man with a thriving practice and a circle of like-minded friends he can still turn like a bear with a sore head, particularly so when he has had a disagreement with one of the faculty.' Johanna turned to Samuel. 'Isn't that the term you use, my dear?' Without waiting for a reply she indicated the young girl next to her. 'Herr Schaefer, you remember Frederika? She has just turned 18 and is already able to hold her own with her cantankerous father.'

Otto Schaefer bowed to the young woman, surprised at how pale she looked, her slight frame in stark contrast to her mother's growing corpulence. 'A pleasure, fraulein.'

Samuel indicated the young man standing beside his wife and daughter. He was a slight man with a shock of black hair that swept back from a clear brow and extended into thick sideburns that bristled above a crisp, white collar.

'Otto, it gives me a great deal of pleasure to introduce Franz Hartmann, one of the brightest young men at the university. Franz had the good sense to give up theology and enrol in medicine. He has also shown himself to be of considerable intellect by attending my lectures each week,' Samuel concluded with a twinkle in his eye.

'But also with enough sense to attend those of the other esteemed professors at the university,' the young man replied.

Schaefer held out his hand to Franz Hartmann. 'It seems you have the measure of our esteemed friend, Herr Hartmann, or should I say our cantankerous friend.'

Hartmann laughed. 'Herr Schaefer, I am far too respectful of Doctor Hahnemann's knowledge and wisdom to take a privilege that only those very close to him would dare voice. But I do not shy away from the conviction that my career can only benefit from exposing myself to all the different teachings and ideas that are available to me at university.'

'And you must never change, Franz,' cried out Samuel Hahnemann. 'I do not entirely reject the teachings of others.' He held out his arms in an exaggerated pose that embraced the room. 'There are many professors far more able than I. Unfortunately we have very few of them here in Leipzig.'

A gentle rumble of laughter filled the room as several of the groups stopped their conversations to welcome the new guest.

'Otto,' Samuel indicated the group nearest them, 'I am being a very poor host.' Schaefer nodded to Hartmann and the two women with a warm smile and followed Samuel.

'Allow me to present Baron Ernst von Brunnow, one of our more sensitive protagonists.'

Schaefer shook hands with the pale youngster. Watery eyes peered at him from above dark smudges.

'Also Doctor Johann Stapf.' Samuel turned and gestured to

the Baron's companion. 'Who, like you, is visiting his old stamping ground.'

'Ah, our esteemed apothecary, it is an honour to meet you, Herr Schaefer. There are not many of your confederacy who are welcome under this roof,' Stapf remarked as he shook hands.

'Perhaps I should be grateful that you did not call it a conspiracy,' Schaefer said, a broad smile taking the sting from his words. 'A union of people created through a common interest, I can live with, plotting evil is another thing entirely.'

'And you do not suspect that some of your fellow pharmacists might not enjoy a little plotting?' The teasing question came from Baron von Brunnow.

'I have no doubt that there are conspirators wherever there is an advantage to be gained by it,' replied Otto, his own smile slipping a trifle.

'I should warn you, Otto,' Samuel interjected, 'you are dealing with a would-be lawyer turned writer who will hear nothing good about the purveyors of allopathy. They have consistently failed to resolve our young baron's health issues. However, he will hear no criticism of those who follow the true faith of homeopathy.' Samuel smiled disarmingly. 'Whilst Doctor Stapf is a master of chemistry and is so besotted with the chemical relationship of natural bodies that he has become my most willing disciple in the proving of new medicines.' Samuel took Otto's arm, steering him away from the two men with a wink, seen by all. 'You will have ample time to best these two, Otto, neither of them could hold a candle to you on military strategy or philosophy.'

'I'm delighted to hear that the conversation around your table does not rest squarely on the principles of homeopathy,' Otto replied.

'Oh, God forbid. I could think of nothing more boring than for this group to waste its entire intellectual worth on the pursuit of something they spend their weekly labour on.'

Two more young men sat in the corner of the drawing room. With them, Otto recognised Samuel's elder daughter, Caroline.

The two men climbed to their feet, a fair-haired man offering his hand to Caroline.

Caroline held her hand out to Herr Schaefer, who bowed his head, clicking his heels as their hands touched.

'It is a pleasure to see you again. I hope, like your sister, you have found the measure of your father? '

Caroline smiled. 'It is a matter of survival Herr Schaefer.'

'Survival?' blustered Samuel, the smile never leaving his face. 'From the sound of you all anyone would think I'm a difficult person to deal with. Yet the truth is, I'm as docile as a lamb.'

'More like mutton,' Caroline observed, the smile on her face broadening by the second.

'I hope none of you gentlemen have the misfortune to be saddled with unappreciative children.' Samuel shook his head sombrely

'Did I overhear the word cantankerous a few moments ago?' Caroline asked.

Otto's smile lit up his face as he joined in. 'Your mother had the temerity to suggest it was a trait of your father's.'

'Enough. How can I possibly expect any respect from my students or my friends if my family poke fun at me in their presence? Even those to whom I have offered treatment and have cured turn upon me when a pretty young woman directs the attack.'

Samuel laid an arm around the shoulders of a fair-haired man whose high colour Otto suspected did not attest to good health. 'This young man, Otto, is Karl Franz, another who switched allegiance from theology to medicine and who has already proven himself to be highly knowledgable in all areas of botany.'

Franz bowed. 'A pleasure, Herr Schaefer.'

'And last but by no means least, Gustav Gross, whose quiet demeanour is often mistaken for a gruff and unapproachable personality. Having said that, I suspect that the man standing before us is destined to be one of the finest homeopaths this country will ever see.'

Otto was surprised to see a blush creep up the man's

somewhat bloated and coarse features. He held out his hand, which Gross shook perfunctorily.

The introductions complete, Samuel caught the eye of his wife, who gave an almost imperceptible nod. 'Ladies, gentlemen, if you are ready? Otto, I wonder if you would accompany Caroline into supper.'

'It would be my pleasure,' he said, extending an arm to the comely young woman, who, he observed, was a slimmer and younger version of her mother.

'So what do you make of my father's collaborators, Herr Schaefer?' Caroline asked quietly.

'Collaborators? My goodness, tonight I have heard talk of missionaries, confederacies and now collaborators.' Otto Schaefer's voice rang with surprise. 'Collaborators against what?'

'Not *against* anything, Herr Schaefer,' Caroline replied, an amused look on her face. 'Everyone you have met here tonight is part of my father's provers union.' She teased him with a smile.

Otto Schaefer returned her smile. 'A prover's union of collaborators? It sounds somewhat sinister and war mongering,' he laughed.

'Perhaps you are right,' Caroline replied, her eyes sparkling. 'I understand you are an admirer of military strategy. You should ask father to explain his tactics and his battle plans because I have no doubt he is engaged in a war. Right now he is very deliberately amassing round him all the resources and allies he will need for a long and, I suspect, bitter campaign.'

39

The table groaned under the weight of food, but otherwise the setting was austere. Large porcelain dishes overflowed with green vegetables and baked potatoes. A bottle of fine wine stood on the table, each person's glass filled with a moderate amount.

Samuel had placed Otto at his right hand. At the far end sat his beloved Elise. Beside Otto sat the youthful Hartmann, deep in conversation with Frederika. Completing their side of the table was the taciturn Gustav Gross, the perfect foil for Johanna's endless chatter.

On Samuel's left, Johann Stapf regaled Karl Franz with von Haller's principle of dividing tissue. Franz listened politely, nodding occasionally at a point made in Stapf's argument, while also tuning one ear to the conversation next to him between Caroline and Ernst von Brunnow, wedged between mother and oldest daughter.

Otto reached for the glass of wine. 'Samuel, I am intrigued. As we walked into dinner your daughter suggested that I should explore your newly acquired interest in warfare, not to mention command strategies and tactics.'

Samuel picked up his own glass and silently toasted his friend. 'I think you must have misunderstood her, Otto, surely she was remarking about your own interest in these things'

'Oh, no you don't, Samuel. My ears heard every word. Caroline referred to your fellow guests as your collaborators, that they are but one plank in your war strategy. Though I'm not exactly sure who the enemy are,' he muttered.

'So my daughter sees my struggle as a war?' Samuel mused to himself. 'Interesting that she would use such an analogy.'

'Perhaps it was my own fascination with the subject that prompted her,' Otto offered, with a gentle smile.

'Perhaps, but nonetheless she makes a valid comparison.'

'Then I would be fascinated to hear your rules of engagement, and your tactical plans.'

Samuel returned his attention to his food, the small portion of rare beef dwarfed by the vegetables piled beside it. He speared a piece of asparagus. 'I must compliment Johanna and my daughters, they have excelled themselves. These vegetables are cooked to perfection, and the beef is truly sublime.'

'My goodness, I think that is the first time I have ever heard you mention food as something other than a fuel to provide energy.' Schaefer sliced a piece of beef and tasted it. Slowly he nodded his head and smiled. 'But you are right, as usual.'

Samuel cast his eyes around the table, a bleak smile on his face. 'Remember Griesslich, Otto?'

'Vividly. I had never realised that a man could be so transparent in his prejudice. I have to admit that watching his antics in that converted church embarrassed me to the point where I felt I should apologise on behalf of all that have willingly embraced allopathy.'

Samuel speared another piece of vegetable from his plate and nodded as he ate it. 'He certainly didn't always trouble himself with the welfare of humanity, and concerned himself too much with the making of money. His appointment to oversee that hospital always reminded me of the moneychangers in the temple.' Carefully Samuel worked a small piece of meat onto his fork. 'But that is not the point of my comment.' Samuel looked up. 'Griesslich reminded me of what I had been fighting against all my life, and he hardened my resolve.'

'Resolve to do what exactly?'

'To ensure that every man, woman and child can expect and receive medical treatment that will give lasting restoration of health, or the removal of the malady in its entirety, in the shortest, most dependable and least harmful way.'

'Perhaps my question should not have been what, but how and who?' Schaefer's reply was touched with a hint of frustration. 'They would be the questions asked by the military strategist. Who is the enemy? Where are they? What is their strength?'

'In many ways the enemy is apathy and ignorance, Otto.' Samuel laid a hand on the sleeve of his friend. 'Unless the populace are aware of what is available to them, how can they make an educated choice? Is that the fault of the medical fraternity, through prejudice, or society in general, through ignorance?'

'Napoleon fought in excess of 300,000 men in the Battle of the Nations and was heavily defeated,' Otto interrupted. 'By your definition you are confronted by an even greater army than the Emperor was.'

'Very true, Otto, but fortunately I don't have cannon and musket raised against me. Just attitudes.' Samuel glanced around, pleased to see that each guest at his table was still engrossed in the conversations of their partners. At the opposite end of the table Johanna leaned back to allow the two young students on either side of her to vigorously debate the importance of translating the *Organon* into French. Samuel caught his wife's eye. She smiled; a contented look on her face.

'Tell me, Otto, what do you believe was Napoleon's true strength as a military strategist?'

'My goodness, where would one start?' Otto rubbed his clean-shaven chin as he considered his response. 'It would be impossible to ignore his capacity to out-think his opponents and, even when heavily outnumbered, spring an attack to catch them by complete surprise.'

'So you would agree that Napoleon clearly understood the strengths and weaknesses of his own forces.'

Otto nodded. 'That is the one thing that could be guaranteed because, unfortunately, he could not always claim the same intimate knowledge of his enemy.'

'I remember you making that very same comment in your study years ago. Until then I had always assumed that Napoleon's intelligence would be faultless.'

'Most people make the same mistake,' Otto replied.

'So his knowledge of his own strengths empowered him to make decisions that could turn looming defeat into victory?' Samuel asked quietly, taking a sip from his wine as he waited for a reply.

'Absolutely.'

'And even when he was licking his wounds, he had the sense to rebuild his army, piece by piece, each block carefully put in its place, a jigsaw that Napoleon could take apart and put back together as his needs dictated.'

'A good analogy, Samuel, although not one I would have used. But what is your point?'

'Please bear with me,' Samuel smiled. He paused to reflect on his next words. 'There is no denying that for many years I gave my opponents every opportunity to weaken my position. Each time I won a battle, I then lost the initiative by withdrawing or casting the victory aside. Call it conceit or pigheadedness, what does it matter now? Even at Molschleben, Otto, my small success over milk scab should have been a victory to build on. Instead I threw the advantage away in the waste of my wanderings.' Samuel again paused in his reflections. 'No, that is too harsh by far. My wanderings served a purpose and I should never deny that.' His reflection over, he rushed on once more. 'It happened again in Königslutter where I battled and defeated scarlet fever.'

'Samuel, you are too harsh by half. Those victories are remembered and acknowledged. Your reputation has survived, whatever damage you think you have done to it.'

'Has it? Certainly my practice is flourishing. Why shouldn't it? I cure people of their maladies. But, you are missing my point entirely. Think of Napoleon. Even in defeat he was always looking at the next round, the next battle. That is what I have always failed to do: build on my successes and make sure I didn't repeat the same mistake.'

'Again, I suspect you are being too generous to Napoleon. Even his last battle at Waterloo was littered with mistakes that he had made before.'

'Then, in what I think may well be my own Waterloo, I will succeed as Wellington and Blücher succeeded, by learning from my mistakes.'

'So, Samuel, I deduce from this that you have already worked out your battle plan?'

'Oh, most assuredly, Otto. I have also selected the generals who will help me win the war.'

Otto looked around the table. Each of the young men was deep in conversation with a colleague. A debate had developed across the table between Hartman, to Otto's right, and Stapf opposite. Young Franz was deep in conversation with Caroline about the latest Paris fashions, while the Baron and Gustav Gross had Johanna enthralled with a story that had nothing to do with medicine.

'That's right,' Samuel's gaze followed the apothecary's, 'these men will be my generals. And between us I believe we can truly win this war.' Samuel smiled benignly at his friend. 'Perhaps generals is too lofty a title, but remember, Otto, you introduced the military analogy.'

'To be precise, it was Caroline,' responded Otto, 'but for the moment I will accept the blame if it brings you to the point of all this.'

'Patience never was your strong suit. Do you recall those lectures of mine that you attended?' Samuel asked.

'Most assuredly. One of my greatest regrets is that I could only attend that first semester before I left for Dresden.'

'So you were not put off by my strange behaviour and antics?'

Otto smiled. 'Eccentric, perhaps, but certainly not strange. I always wondered how you coped with some of the younger students smirking and twittering behind your back.'

'Better than the sneering and condemnation my so-called peers brought to the lectures. Anyway, don't you remember your first terms at university? How many years ago was that?' Samuel asked innocently.

'Your sense of humour gets worse by the year. And stop changing the subject. You are, I swear, the most frustrating person to talk to.'

'Calm down. If you don't want to answer my perfectly innocent question, I shall remind you. A pre-requisite of every young man's entry into university is an empty mind and a sense of fun and adventure that often borders on the crude, but the mind must always be open and willing.'

Otto laughed quietly at his friend's description.

'Which part tickles you most? My description of their empty minds or your own memory at some of the pranks you played on your fellows or, God forbid, the faculty.'

'Both ... all of them ... just as your sly tactics anticipated.'

Samuel assumed a serious demeanour. 'My point,' he continued, 'is that most, if not all, of the qualified doctors in this city have disowned me and my theories.' He fluttered a hand in dismissal. 'Anyway, most of them are too lazy or too busy making money to go back to school and learn something new.'

'There you go again. Every time you speak about your peers you put them down. Why should they respect you?' Otto shook his head in despair.

'An interesting conundrum, Otto.' Samuel smiled across at Doctor Stapf who was listening with keen interest to the exchange between Samuel and Otto.

'I am the first to admit that my theories are a long way from being completely vindicated, but there is a mounting testimony of proof that homeopathy works. The smart way to ensure it has a chance to grow and prosper is through the minds and energies of young people who are not closed to new ideas.'

'For the first time since this conversation began I find myself in complete agreement with you, and I also think I am beginning to see your strategy.'

'Thank goodness!' Samuel slapped the heel of his palm against his forehead. 'Then perhaps we should withdraw to the other room where I can have a pipe and you can explain to me how Napoleon would have achieved the same goals.'

40

Samuel tamped down the tobacco. Carefully he struck a match and held it over the bowl as he drew the smoke deep. He and Otto sat in a large alcove surrounded on three sides by large ornate windows. They had a clear view of the evening's company through a wide archway.

'That is why I deemed it necessary to establish a clear strategy to recruit people who would take us forward.' Samuel drew on his pipe and surveyed the drawing room. 'Two of the young men at dinner came to me for medical reasons. I will not break any confidences but both of them had reached a point of despair with their current treatment. And each of them has found significant relief, if not a complete cure through homeopathy. Like the others they are brilliant students with enquiring minds.'

Otto nodded. 'I think I understand,' his brow creased, 'and if I am right, your tactics included the oblique reference you made to your appearance at those lectures I attended?'

'Many things are contrived, Otto, even things that may appear otherwise.'

'You're saying that you deliberately played up to your audience?'

'Absolutely. Do you really believe I was naïve enough to think I could convert my critics, who, as you so kindly reminded me, have been on the receiving end of most of my invective?'

'And these gatherings?' Otto asked indicating the company.

'The same. But there is nothing contrived about our affections or our commitment to these young men. I have been very candid with each of them. At worst I could be accused of waiting to see which way they would lean, but,' Samuel shrugged his shoulders, 'surely even Napoleon employed such tactics in selecting his own generals?'

'But once selected he would have given his generals his complete confidence.'

'As I have mine,' Samuel replied. 'Do not underestimate my determination. Every one of the men in this house understands perfectly the importance of establishing homeopathy and what is required to do so. Each one of them is as motivated as I am, having already experienced the hatred and derision of our enemies.'

'My goodness, Samuel, you truly have developed a sense for the dramatic. What have these young men done to incur such enemies apart from attending your lectures? After all, surely that is why they attend university — to learn.'

'And learn what?' Blue smoke poured out from Samuel's mouth and nostrils, forming a cloud around his head. Don't you see that is exactly my point? Not one of these young men was satisfied with what they were being told. They questioned their professors until the good men of allopathy threw their hands in the air. But did they change their methods to satisfy these enquiring minds?' Samuel shook his head disturbing the layer of smoke. 'No, of course they didn't. Each one of these men is a true scholar, with the driving ambition of scholars to be part of the process not merely the object of it.' More smoke poured from Samuel's pipe until the air around the two men was blue. Samuel took the pipe from his mouth and waved it at the different groups. 'Ask them. Ask these young people whether I have abused their trust or whether they have agreed willingly. In fact it is they who have pushed these ideas even further than I was prepared to do.'

'I don't think I have ever suggested that you have abused

their trust,' Otto said.

'I'm sorry to interrupt, Herr Schaefer.' Franz Hartmann stood above the two men. 'We have learnt from experience that when the smoke signals start to go up, one of our guests needs to be rescued.' The youngster smiled and then pulled up a chair.

'Tell this heretic what Clarus has decreed,' Samuel beamed through the clearing smoke, and then turned to Otto. 'You do remember Clarus? Excuse me ... I should have said professor, Professor Doctor Clarus, the esteemed clinical professor at the University of Leipzig.'

Otto nodded while sharing a conspiratorial smile with young Hartmann.

'Our esteemed dictator,' Hartmann added then turned to his mentor. 'Not so much what he has decreed, doctor, more what he has inferred.' He turned back to address the apothecary. 'Last week Doctor Clarus took me aside to warn me that he'd had enough of the "carrying's on" of Hahnemann and his pupils.' Hartmann smiled as Otto raised an eyebrow. 'Oh trust me, Professor Clarus makes no bones of his hatred for everything Doctor Hahnemann espouses. Other students hear him calling us "ignorant fellows", which of course they pick up and taunt us with.'

'I'm sorry, but I find this all very ... difficult to understand,' Otto replied, 'It must make it untenable for you to study.'

'The only way to survive is to attend the lectures of other professors, even though most of us find them of little value,' Hartmann added.

Through the smoky haze another man loomed above them. Doctor Stapf pulled a chair forward to join the group. 'I apologise for my interruption, but it is difficult not to overhear, and it would appear that nothing seems to have changed at my old school.'

'Johann, you are always welcome, especially as we are breaking one of our firmest rules.' Samuel waved his pipe at the newcomer.

'And what rule, pray tell, are we breaking,' Otto asked while nodding politely to the newcomer.

'To avoid homeopathy at these dinners.'

Otto started to apologise but Samuel would have none of it. 'I knew from the outset that we would break the rule tonight, Otto. Homeopathy needs friends.'

'You know that I have been a strong supporter for many years, Samuel, even though I suspected that you might ultimately take business from me.' Otto's mouth twisted into a wry smile.

'It is a pity that so many of your colleagues feel threatened by change. Many doctors, like Stapf here, have become converts because they have seen the results for themselves.'

'Unfortunately, Herr Schaefer,' Stapf cut in gently, 'it is the establishment ...'

Playfully Samuel poked the air with his pipe. 'See, Otto, there is that word again. We cannot escape it.'

'The one thing you can always be sure of, Herr Schaefer,' Stapf smiled, persisting with the good natured banter, 'is that the good doctor's dinner parties will always be humorous. Wit rather than wisdom seems to be the order for most.'

'I take exception, Stapf,' Samuel cried. 'Wisdom abounds! Between us, Otto and I must have more than a century of the stuff.'

The room convulsed into laughter. Even those not attending the immediate group paused in their conversations as the cloud of smoke belched forth.

'That's more like it,' Samuel applauded, wiping the tears from his eyes. 'Now you have my permission to resume some of the serious stuff. At least we have had a good laugh.'

'The truth is, Herr Schaefer,' remarked Stapf dryly, 'anyone prepared to learn about homeopathy comes to understand that it is simply part of the balance of things. I studied medicine under Clarus and Rosenmüller. If you know both men you will be aware of their strict adherence to the history of our profession.' Otto nodded silently as Stapf continued. 'It pains me to say this but I took little satisfaction from their dissertations on the history of diseases or their view of the origins of each disease.

Unfortunately, I found myself constantly questioning their theories and their claims. Some of it held up to scrutiny, other parts didn't. Either something was missing in what they taught, or I was striving for something that did not exist. Perhaps it is my preponderance to individualise and observe for myself, but whatever the reason ...' Stapf shrugged his shoulders. 'Have you read the *Organon*, Herr Schaefer?' Stapf asked.

'Yes, Samuel sent me a copy, which, much to the horror of my colleagues, has pride of place on my bookshelf.'

Stapf smiled. 'I first read of the principle of *similia similibus* in my early studies. If my memory serves it was in *Fragmenta de viribus*.'

'My goodness, Stapf, I had that published in 1805; it's almost ancient history,' Samuel interjected.

Stapf smiled at Otto Schaefer, an indulgent look on his face.

'In my early studies I found it very hard to give due credence to Doctor Hahnemann's theories,' Stapf continued blithely. 'Maybe a year before I took my bachelor's examination I acquired a copy of the *Organon*. At first I was sceptical, but I forced myself to study the principles in it. I became entranced by Doctor Hahnemann's view of the pathology of diseases, which was so different to that espoused by Clarus.'

Otto was captivated by the young doctor sitting beside him. Other members of the group had gathered around them, some standing, others sitting on the floor. No doubt they have heard this story before, Otto thought, yet each one appeared entranced by the doctor's easy story-telling, his hold over them powerful yet subtle. Otto smiled to himself, honoured to be in the company of Samuel Hahnemann and his generals.

'I was one of a handful of students who was prepared to think for themselves,' Stapf said. 'Unfortunately Clarus and Rosenmüller breed medical students to follow the safe path.'

A chuckle went up around the group, which Stapf ignored. 'Somewhere, there is the perfect medical solution, one that strikes a natural balance or a natural unity. It pained me to sit in lecture rooms and listen to these academics pontificate on matters that seemed most learned and yet were merely hot air.' Stapf looked around the group, something close to theatrical surprise on his face, as if he were unaware of the audience that had gathered.

Almost reluctantly he resumed. 'Whatever the ambition of the establishment, I find it hard to believe that any of them are truly concerned about the health of the patients they are proposing to treat. Rather, they are encouraged to consider what others will think of them, to not deviate from the standard in case they be criticised for breaking convention.'

'Bravo, Doctor Stapf,' cried Samuel Hahnemann. 'How eloquently you expand my inadequate theories. And how sad that the very core of our society constantly rejects change because they are frightened that, through it, they will lose, not gain.'

41

The portly middle-aged apothecary and the quixotic young doctor left together. By chance both were staying at the small inn just off the Burgstrasse, where Otto and Samuel had once reflected on the death of the apothecary's son.

'I enjoyed my sojourn here in Leipzig,' Stapf remarked to his companion, 'but I am always happy to be able to return to my home.'

'Where is home, doctor?'

'I was born in Naumberg, my father is pastor of the Maria Magdalena Church there.'

'Have you always lived there, except for your time here in Leipzig?'

Stapf shook his head. 'At eleven, my father and mother sent me to Porta. But after three years my mother became alarmed at the deterioration in my health and insisted I return home.' Stapf smiled. 'Now I suspect I will spend my life there.'

'And continue your work as one of Samuel's collaborators?'

'I prefer the term provers, Herr Schaefer. But, yes, like collaborators. Doctor Hahnemann argued that unless we worked together to prove our principles we would continue to be exposed to scorn and ridicule.'

'I was surprised at the comment by young Hartmann that

the faculty persecuted Samuel's students.'

'Not surprising when you consider that Clarus is not only the clinical professor at the university, but is also the highest medical authority in Saxony. If he so desired he could set himself up as judge and jury and get away with it. No student could risk attending only Doctor Hahnemann's lectures, a bitter pill that our good doctor has been forced to swallow.'

Otto grinned at the irony in the pun, but Stapf had serious matters on his mind and the humour quickly evaporated.

'You know Doctor Hahnemann as well, if not better, than any of us, Herr Schaefer,' he said in the shadowy light cast by the oil lamps, 'so you would well-understand that such a pill would only serve as a catalyst for the good doctor to plot against the bearer.'

'Yes, the more he observed the petty antics of Clarus, the more determined he would be to bring about change.'

'Exactly. And he went about it by following the oldest rule of pedagogy, whereby the true scholar is not content with instruction but wants to be an integral part of the lesson.'

'And the proving of Samuel's theories would be a logical place for the students to start,' added Schaefer.

Stapf agreed. 'With students who were already convinced that the only way forward for medicine was in the pursuit of homeopathy.'

'Surely most were too young and inexperienced to be able to make such an absolute decision?' Otto asked, his voice unable to hide his astonishment.

'Doctor Hahnemann cured Franz Hartmann of a particularly difficult ailment, one that everyone else had given up on,' Stapf said. 'von Brunnow was plagued with several ailments, including particular problems with his eyes. He had completely lost faith in the medical fraternity, until he was introduced to Doctor Hahnemann.'

'So,' Otto's words dripped with scorn, 'I'm hearing that Samuel's cures are at the heart of this ... this overwhelming conviction that miracles are possible and they can transform homeopathy into the shining light for the future of the world. Is that correct, Doctor Stapf, or do my ears deceive me?'

'Your cynicism does you no credit, Herr Schaefer.'

'Excuse me, Doctor Stapf,' Otto spluttered at the sharpness in Stapf's voice, 'I don't think it is my cynicism that should be on trial here but the smugness of my companion. I listened to you speak in Samuel's home and admired your ability to persuade others with your story. But you are naïve in the extreme if you think that average, well-meaning folk will accept such a simple proposition.'

Stapf felt his face burning. 'Had Doctor Hahnemann not advocated your independence on these matters I would be forced to assume your prejudices matched those of all apothecaries, most of whom make even Professor Clarus appear pure and pristine.'

'Ah, so now we are at the nub of it,' Otto said quietly. 'Sir, you are a very impressive man. Your conviction and your passion do you enormous credit. There are not many men who impress me so on first meeting them. But I fear that your prejudices are as difficult to shift as those of other men. Even though my good friend has vouched for my tolerance you truly find it hard to believe that an apothecary could be open-minded.'

Stapf stopped walking, causing Otto to follow suit. A chill had settled around the city, the night sky above them sparkled with stars. Otto pulled his topcoat tighter, trapping the warmth to his ample girth as he waited for his companion to choose his words.

'I apologise if I appeared rude, Herr Schaefer,' Stapf said formally. 'You are right, I don't trust the apothecaries. The ridicule and persecution visited on the students by Clarus and his cronies is also a way of life in my practice, courtesy of the pharmacists. Even though I am qualified in allopathy, I practice only homeopathy, which leaves me exposed to the infantile and often defamatory mischief of the apothecaries in Naumberg.'

'I wasn't seeking an apology, doctor.' Otto replied contritely. 'I inflamed the situation by not biting my tongue and allowing you to finish.'

Stapf inclined his head and indicated to his companion that they resume the short walk to their accommodation. 'I should not have been so emphatic about the student's conviction towards homeopathy or appear to suggest that they should not pay due diligence to the other disciplines. But nor should we underestimate how perceptive Doctor Hahnemann has been and how influential the simple act of inviting students to participate in proving our remedies is in gaining their ultimate loyalty.'

'It is late,' Otto Schaefer observed as the entrance to the inn appeared, illuminated by a flickering oil lamp. 'I have heard a great deal about this business of proving. Tomorrow I have been invited to join Samuel and some of his young colleagues in a discussion on new remedies. If it would not be too much of an imposition I would be grateful for your guidance as to what might transpire. Perhaps we could meet over breakfast?'

A little before eight Otto joined Johann Stapf in the dining room of the small inn. The doctor had already given his order to the daughter of the innkeeper.

Otto rubbed his hands together. 'Doctor Stapf, I hope you slept well. I know I did! Thoughts of the breakfast our gracious innkeeper's wife provides sent me to sleep with blissful dreams.'

'Then I'm sad to be the bearer of unpleasant news,' Doctor Stapf said, a solemn expression on his face.

'What?' Otto looked around at the kitchen door through which the young waitress had disappeared. 'Don't tell me she's not here this morning.'

Schaefer turned back to Stapf, who was slowly shaking his head.

'Oh my goodness, what could have happened?' Otto blurted out.

Stapf let out a laugh, a broad smile creasing his face. 'I'm sorry, Herr Schaefer, but your face was so serious, I couldn't resist.'

An embarrassed look touched Otto Schaefer's brow. 'Very unfair, Doctor Stapf. I am a man of few vices; unfortunately one of them is food.' Otto smiled at his colleague.

Their conversation was interrupted by the reappearance of the young girl. Otto ran a hand over his freshly shaven jowls, his eyes peering heavenward for inspiration. He gave his order and sweetly requested the young girl to repeat it back to him.

Stapf tried to keep a smile from his face and steered the conversation between Otto's hunger pangs; the apothecary being distracted throughout the exchange.

'I would assume that Doctor Hahnemann has spoken to you of the remedies that he has used as the basis for his theories. When he wrote the *Organon* there were twenty-six medicines that he had proven to his own satisfaction.'

The door to the kitchen swung open. Stapf paused as the waitress rested a massive tray on the edge of the table and began piling food in front of Otto Schaefer. Small dishes of pickles jostled with plates laden with cold meats and boiled eggs. A basket of small, sweet rolls joined the rest, small curls of golden butter scooped into a bowl in the midst of them. The young girl wiped her brow with the hem of her apron and placed a single plate with several sweet rolls and an apple in front of Stapf.

Otto Schaefer eyed the meagre offerings in front of his companion and then cast a protective gaze over his own fare. 'Should I get the girl back with something more substantial?' he asked, pointing at Stapf's plate.

'I'm very content, thank you, Herr Schaefer.' Stapf struggled to keep the smile from his face and began to slice the apple with a sharp knife. 'Perhaps I should continue my explanation.' Otto simply nodded and continued buttering a sweet roll.

'Proving the original twenty-six remedies was a massive undertaking for one man,' Stapf said. 'For Doctor Hahnemann to take the next step on his own was not practical. He needed assistance, but not just from healthy volunteers who were prepared to subject themselves to the testing of drugs on their own bodies. What he really needed was a group of like-minded scholars who could conduct the research in such a manner that it was irrefutable.'

Otto Schaefer swallowed a portion of sweet roll slathered with butter and heaped with cold pork. 'Isn't this paranoia going a little too far, Doctor Stapf?' He lifted the corner of his napkin and wiped away a dribble of butter from his chin. 'No-one has demanded such diligence for the medicines on my shelves?'

'Interesting that you should use paranoia and diligence in the same breath, Herr Schaefer. Like Doctor Hahnemann, I regard diligence as essential if we are to break new ground. On the other hand, paranoia is a state of mind usually observed by those who are uncomfortable with the likely outcome.'

'Stapf, please, don't play word games with me at breakfast. I'm only a mere apothecary; I can concentrate on only one thing at a time.'

Stapf ignored the sally. 'Your earlier point is well-made. When I was studying under Clarus and his cronies I was taught that for centuries doctor's had worked according to precedent. Anyone who understands the principals of homeopathy will see the flaws in blindly accepting precedent. Just because the old masters swore by a certain medicine to treat a certain symptom does not make it right.'

'Why should they need to question it?'

'I would remind you of the basic precept of homeopathy, Herr Schaefer. Unlike what the old masters were doing, we are not treating the disease or the single set of symptoms. We are adamant that the problem is much more deeply rooted than its superficial manifestation. Therefore, the giving of medicine to treat one symptom must be assessed on the effect it will have on the whole. Clearly it is the duty of the physician to distinguish the subtleties of every single patient.'

'Am I to assume that you are saying one medicine, correctly identified, will cure a patient of all their ills, not just the ailment that has brought them to the doctor in the first place?' Otto Schaefer mumbled through a mouthful of egg.

'In its crudest form, yes. And it is the responsibility of every homeopathic physician to distinguish the subtle variations within every patient.'

'In every case?'

'To simply acknowledge the symptoms of a disease and treat them with a known remedy is not only lazy, it is negligent. How does the physician know what other problems lurk in the body and, thereby, the danger the prescribed medicine could be doing elsewhere?'

'In such a case,' replied Otto, 'the physician would simply prescribe a second treatment to deal with the problem.'

'And then a third or, God forbid, even a fourth?' Stapf remarked dryly.

'Well,' Otto Schaefer hesitated, 'well, yes, if necessary. We've been dispensing more than one medicine to patients for years. Not many of them die, for goodness sake.'

'The only thing that is proven about the drugs you dispense from your pharmacy, Herr Schaefer, is that they will deal with the symptoms of the malaise. There is nothing proven about them that says they will cure the patient.'

'But what you are suggesting would require the identification of thousands of symptoms ...'

'And the accurate recording of those symptoms,' Stapf added, 'Along with a detailed description of how each proven medicine would assist with those symptoms in each individual.'

'That is a massive, painstaking undertaking, Doctor Stapf,' Otto Schaefer said in quiet amazement. And you believe that through your provings you can change the establishment?'

'I am convinced of it, Herr Schaefer. We have already seen proof of it in the success of Doctor Hahnemann's practice — even in my own, in a small way. People come back because our remedies work'

'But surely it's impractical to think that you can test every medicine in your lifetime. Certainly not in Samuel's.'

'The very enormity of the task is why there is a need for a group of collaborators who will be disciplined enough to follow the procedure Doctor Hahnemann has stipulated.'

'To make the results verifiable?'

'So you do have knowledge of research protocol, Herr

Schaefer.' Stapf teased. 'Yes, absolutely, to ensure the results will stand up to any scrutiny. In the early days, Doctor Hahnemann supplied the medicines to each of us in the form of an essence or a tincture, always ensuring we understood the genesis of the medicine.'

'I am cautious not to overreact as I did last night, but surely this is a very dangerous game you are describing?' Otto had forgotten about the scraps still in front of him and was listening with increasing interest.

'Invariably he had already tried the drugs on himself so he had some sense of what strength we should take.' Stapf smiled. 'I remember one of the first letters I received from Doctor Hahnemann after I had returned to Naumberg. The instructions were meticulous. He described exactly how many drops should be placed in exactly how much water. Even the strength of the tincture he had provided was noted, to ensure no-one tried to deviate from the discipline. Then the instructions detailed how many drops to take, how often and when. And, as if these precautions were not enough, he always included a suggested remedy that would allay the symptoms should they become too severe.'

'Now I know we are talking about my friend,' Otto said, an indulgent smirk on his face.

Stapf returned the smile. 'Oh it doesn't end there, Herr Schaefer. Each of his current collaborators is required to provide a detailed response in the form of a lengthy screed where they enter up their observations of the symptoms they experience, at what time of day and in what circumstances.'

'I'm not sure I follow.'

'Doctor Hahnemann insists that every one of us should follow a strict routine. He forbids the use of coffee, tea or other substances, even spices and salted food, anything that may influence the symptoms he is looking for.'

'Not even in the lifetime of your children,' Otto Schaefer muttered, shaking his head in disbelief.

'I'm sorry?' Stapf said, looking up from the debris in front of the apothecary.

'I made some facetious remark about the amount of work involved. Clearly I underestimated.' Otto waved his hand in the air. 'This is fascinating, Doctor Stapf, please don't let me interrupt you.'

'Doctor Hahnemann now insists that we provide the medicinal substances ourselves, especially the herbal ones.'

'Surely Samuel had his reasons.'

'Most definitely. In this way each of the collaborators became familiar with the changes that take place in the materials used to make the medicines. Simple things such as the change in the seasons have the potential to affect the efficacy of the cure.'

'I had no idea of the complexity or the level of commitment all of you have made to your profession.' Otto reached into his pocket and took out his fob watch. 'My goodness, it is already well past nine. My sincere apologies, sir, if I have kept you from your business.'

Johann Stapf smiled and shook his head. 'My work is at the university library, I am not keeping anyone waiting but myself. But what of you?'

Otto Schaefer climbed to his feet. 'I am due to attend a meeting with the local society of apothecaries. Several of the university's esteemed medical faculty will be there.' Otto smiled as Stapf raised an eyebrow. 'I'm not sure if the celebrated Professor Clarus is one of them. The apothecaries are proposing to discuss their future in this beloved country of ours. They are not so blind that they cannot see things are changing. Of interest will be what they resolve to do given the increasing interest being shown to homeopathy by the public. I will be very surprised if the meeting can reach its completion without some mention of Samuel Hahnemann.'

42

Thirty men were crowded into the small upstairs room of the inn a short distance past the university.

Otto recognised several of them from his time in Leipzig. Others were newcomers or had travelled in from the outlying villages and towns where they conducted their practices. A tall, heavy-set man whose dark hair was laced with streaks of grey tapped him on the shoulder.

'Albert Wagner, my goodness it must be more than twenty years?' Otto Schaefer held out his hand to the newcomer. 'Last I heard, you'd moved from Stotteritz and settled in Berlin.'

The big man acknowledged Otto with a nod. 'Moved in '94. An opportunity to expand came up through family connections.' Albert Wagner leaned closer. 'Truth is I could never have lasted at Stotteritz — too many small-minded people — on the other hand, Berlin!' Wagner's eyes lit up. 'Ah, what can one say about Berlin? Except for the Prussians, the city is almost perfect. The theatre there is a miracle ... the restaurants ... well, how can you describe them? The only word adequate enough is sublime. The place is positively vibrant. Don't tell me you haven't found it so?'

'Never been.' Otto replied, the expression on his face deliberately blank. 'Always seemed to be too busy, and now that I've moved down to Dresden, I'm even further away.'

'Dresden, eh? Has the place recovered from the beating the little Corsican gave it?'

'Fortunately much of that battle occurred in the countryside,' Otto said warily, conscious that the man's arrogance had not changed one scintilla since their university days together. 'So have you left the wonders of Berlin behind you, or are you planning to return?'

'Left for good, I'm afraid.' A dark curtain drew across Wagner's eyes. 'My wife lost her mother after a long illness a year or so back. The good lady decided she needed to be close to her during that difficult time.'

'So back to Stotteritz?'

'Oh, goodness me, no,' the big man boomed. 'We live here in Leipzig. With the profit from Berlin I was more than able to afford the necessary coachman and the finest Landau. My wife travelled the three miles there and back in supreme comfort.'

Otto was saved by a loud call from the front of the room.

'Gentlemen, if I could please ask everyone to find a seat.'

Otto looked around, trying to find the source of the instruction. Two hands waved above the milling crowd. Finally several of the apothecaries at the front of the room sat down, revealing the chairman. He was a short man, no more than five feet tall, wearing a black suit, well cut, his short legs cloaked in white hose, the same colour as the mass of curls on his head. His polished black shoes jumped up and down as he strained to see the back of the room over the heads of the people still standing. Behind the chairman two men made their way to seats arranged on the small dais. Otto grinned when he recognised Clarus.

Taking Wagner's elbow, Otto indicated a pair of chairs that had been left empty on the end of the third row. 'Let's claim those two before some other enterprising pharmacists do.'

At the front of the room the chairman appeared to be gaining the upper hand, the noise in the small room dropping a couple of notches as the audience concentrated on finding a seat. At last the diminutive chairman had a clear view over the heads of the assembled members.

'Gentlemen, as you all know... Gentlemen, please.' He waved his hands one final time. The room fell silent. 'Thank goodness.' The chairman wiped a sleeve across his brow and took a deep breath. 'All of you are aware of the reason why this meeting was called.' He looked around the room waiting for someone to challenge him. Every man in the room stared back.

He continued. 'There is a growing disquiet amongst some of our members, er ... which I understand is shared by some of the medical fraternity and university faculty.' He turned his head to acknowledge the two men seated behind him. 'Some of them believe that, er, that some of the newer modalities ...'

'Get to the point, Beck.' The shout came from a florid-faced man sitting towards the back of the room. 'They call it homeopathy, if you can't pronounce it.'

Otto Schaefer turned in his seat to get a clearer view of the man who had interjected. Slowly he turned back to face the front, a sense of disquiet growing in his stomach.

On the dais, Herr Beck's face flushed the same colour as that of his antagonist. He waited for the murmur of approval from the audience to quieten. 'I'm perfectly capable of pronouncing it, Herr Schlutt,' the chairman said stiffly, 'and I suggest for the moment that we display a sense of propriety until we have discussed the agenda for this meeting.'

'That is the bloody agenda, Beck,' his antagonist called out. 'That's why you were instructed to invite Professor Clarus, so we could gain a clearer view of the university's position. Let's get on with it.'

Another chorus of approval swelled throughout the gathering, while beads of perspiration formed on the chairman's forehead.

'Gentlemen, please. 'At least have the courtesy to allow me to finish the introductions.'

'Hooray,' came the cry from another part of the room.

'And hurry up about it,' the florid faced man rejoined. 'At least then we can listen to some intelligent debate.'

Otto leant towards Albert Wagner. 'Not a very popular

chairman,' he observed in a soft voice.

Wagner's smile was bleak. 'This is mild compared to some of the meetings I've attended,' he whispered back.

On the small dais, the chairman was sweating profusely, muttering to himself while pulling a handkerchief from his sleeve. Beck mopped his brow and then returned the handkerchief. From his pocket he took out a folded page. He cleared his throat.

'Er ... Professor Clarus, um ... you all know Professor Clarus, the clinical professor at the university, and ... er, medical councillor. With Professor Clarus is Professor Dzondi, who is, um ... visiting the university from Halle.' The chairman appeared to gain some inspiration from the words on his sheet of paper. 'Some of you may already be familiar with Professor Dzondi from his letters and articles that are appearing in our presses. We have extended an invitation to both men to join us today to ...'

'We know why, Beck.' Again it was the florid-faced man at the back of the room. 'We want to know whether we should be getting concerned about this business or whether it's just another flash in the pan. Ever since the little Corsican General ran with his tail between his legs, the newspapers have been looking for some excitement to fill their front pages. And for a while they found it, courtesy of Hahnemann's luck in the typhus scare.'

Otto went very still at the mention of Samuel's name. The agenda was becoming very pointed.

Sensing the impending disaster, Professor Clarus rose to his feet and stepped to the front of the small dais. His face was pale, made even starker by the shock of dark hair that he swept back with his hand as he approached the chairman. His eyes sparked as he surveyed the room.

'Allow me to answer the gentleman's concern, Herr Beck.' The words were silky, chilling, the famed academic correctly reading the mood of the room. Clarus pulled himself to his full height, his medium stature towering over the diminutive chairman.

'It would be wrong of me to say that I understand the predilections of the editors of our fair presses,' Clarus said to the waiting audience, a thin smile on his lips, 'but I echo the concern of our friend at the back. Whenever the press are without a juicy story they go looking for one or, dare I say it, conjure one up from some mischief that is fed to them by some self-serving opportunist.'

'Hear, hear. We should be looking to do the same,' the florid-faced man interjected, bringing a wider smile to the face of the professor.

Clarus held up his hands. 'Allow me to state the position of the university.' Clarus paused and surveyed the room. 'Dean Ludwig and, before him, Rösenmuller, were prepared to embrace new teachings and new ideas. To not do so would be contrary to everything that we hold as the core purpose of our charter. But to acknowledge the need is not to blindly accept what comes from it. And that, gentlemen, is something I will certainly never do.'

'Good to hear,' cried out Albert Wagner, making Otto jump. Around him a chorus of voices picked up the cry.

On the dais, Clarus beamed at the assembled group and then stole a glance behind him at his colleague, smirking, allowing the noise to wear itself out before continuing. 'Those of you who know me know of my passion for precedent. Our forefathers have diligently documented very good reasons why the medicines they prescribe should continue.'

'But not substantive proof,' Otto muttered to himself under his breath.

Blithely unaware of any interruption Professor Clarus kept talking.

'The weight of history is on the side of these eminently qualified men who for centuries have been prescribing the drugs you dispense. Yet the so-called homeopathic modality that Hahnemann espouses has criticised these drugs, claiming, amongst other contentions, that they are prescribed in unnecessary quantities and, even more to the point, that they are suppressive.'

'Maybe we should suppress him,' interjected the florid-faced man.

Clarus nodded sagely at the interruption and waited for the noise to subside. 'Not long ago, my colleagues attended one of Hahnemann's lecture in which he made the astonishing claim that the drugs you dispense simply mask the person's symptoms, creating deeper, more serious diseases.' Clarus shook his head.

'Kick him out of the university; it's bloody heresy,' a tall man at the back of the room shouted.

Clarus held up his hands, careful to hide the smile forming on his lips. 'As I said, it is the highest duty of the university to foster new thinking, new ideas. No-one, including me, would challenge that charter, but that does not mean I condone what is being spruiked.'

'Hear, hear,' went up the chant around the room.

'It is clearly a ludicrous situation,' Clarus opined. 'In the same breath, these homeopaths claim that this so-called masking of symptoms makes it more difficult for them, ultimately, to find the correct medicine, so they seek to invent their own.' Clarus stood in front of his audience shaking his head in mute disbelief.

'You may not be aware that I have placed a ban on students attending Doctor Hahnemann's lectures at the exclusion of others. As of now, anyone who does not look at all aspects of the medical sciences will not pass their bachelor exam. Gentlemen, you have my word on that.'

A cheer went up in the small room. Professor Clarus waited for the noise to quieten before holding out an arm. 'My colleague, Professor Dzondi, is burning up with impatience to tell his story.' Clarus paused theatrically, allowing his words to sink in. 'All of you will have seen Hahnemann's outrageous attack in the press on Professor Dzondi's advocacy for the perfectly legitimate treatment for burns. Using cold water has been advocated for centuries under the premise of *contraria contrariis*. Not only does the good professor support the premise, he has undertaken experiments on himself to prove them. I should also add that he has written a small book on the matter, which I'm sure he will gladly sell to you for a few groschen to ensure that your customers can have the value of his wisdom.'

Otto clamped a hand to his mouth to stop himself from laughing out loud, hiding his disbelief at the barefaced temerity of the man behind a paroxysm of sneezing and coughing.

Clarus threw a glance in Otto's direction before returning to his compliant audience. 'Please welcome the good professor from Halle, who will tell you in his own words how false Hahnemann's accusations are, and how the truth is being distorted. The good professor is so confident of his position that he has challenged Doctor Hahnemann to a bet of 500 gold thaler to prove which is the better cure. A bet, I would point out, that Hahnemann has refused to accept.'

Clarus and Dzondi stayed briefly to share some refreshments with the apothecaries before departing and leaving in their wake a restless audience whose beliefs had been inflamed by their rhetoric. From the dais, the chairman was waving his arms, attempting to be heard above the angry buzz.

Otto slumped back into his seat, hoping to encourage an end to the sordid assembly. Slowly, others took their seats until only a small group of men remained standing, their argument giving no appearance of abating. Otto identified the florid-faced man and his tall companion from the back of the room. Also among the group was Albert Wagner.

'Gentlemen, if you will resume your seats, please.' The chairman directed his entreaty towards the group. 'If you sit down we can move to a resolution.' The group made no attempt to break up, apparently oblivious to anything except their anger.

'Rhinehart, Wagner, get a move on. Come on, Schlutt, I've got a bloody council to run.' A burly man with heavy mutton-chops shouted above the chairman. Otto turned to inspect the man, only a few seats from him.

'C'mon, get on with it. I haven't got all day,' the man called out.

Reluctantly the small group broke up, scowls etched on each man's face as they resumed their seats. The burly man then turned to Herr Beck. 'Now get on with it, Beck. Let's get a motion on the table and be done with it.'

'Hear, hear,' echoed the apothecaries around the room.

'Thank you, Doctor Volkmann,' the chairman said. 'Is there anyone who wishes to propose a motion from the floor?'

A hand shot up from the side of the room furthest from Otto Schaefer, his view of the man blocked by six or seven bodies.

'What really sticks in my gullet,' the new speaker opined, 'is that these people are becoming too popular by half. If it keeps going I'll be a pauper before the decade's done. They don't necessarily break any laws, to give them their due, but it's this confounded dosage business. How can anyone make any money with the piddling quantities these homopathies hand out?'

'Homeopaths,' Otto blurted out before he could stop himself.

'Whatever,' replied the man, making no attempt to eyeball who had corrected him. 'Then they only recommend one medicine at a time. How's a man to make any money when they claim one remedy is all that is needed to fix a patient's ills?'

'I agree! And too much bloody work by half,' another man interjected. 'Each time a patient comes in with a prescription from one of those fellows it takes me double the time to prepare it. One time one of the fool homeopaths even came into the shop and accused me of making up the wrong remedy.'

'I can't see what your problem is.' The call came from the back of the room where a tall, aesthetic blond man rose to his feet. 'There's a whole group of us who've never even had one of them in our shops. We reckon you're blowing this thing right out of proportion. Even if it does catch on, how many d'you reckon there'll be, twenty, thirty? And I mean in the whole of Saxony, not just here in Leipzig.'

'Gentlemen.' This time it was Beck calling from the front of the room. 'Gentlemen, if we don't get a motion on the table soon I fear we will all miss our lunch. Is anyone prepared to move a motion?'

'Yes, I say we should lobby the university to stop

Hahnemann's lectures. He's just inciting trouble.' The call came from the man Volkmann had identified as Rhinehart.

'No matter what Clarus says,' Doctor Volkmann replied, 'the university won't stop Doctor Hahnemann from lecturing. And even if they did, there is nothing in our rules that would prevent Doctor Hahnemann from establishing his own college.'

'Excuse me, sir,' Otto interjected, directing his words to Doctor Volkmann, 'I'm a visitor from Dresden. What are these rules you speak of?'

'The council ordinances. There's nothing in our regulations that prevent such a college from being established. Nor does the state have any such rule. Not to mention that it would be a massive undertaking to persuade our king to be so bold or radical,' Volkmann replied.

'You are obviously very well-informed, sir. Can I ask what your role is in all this? I presumed you were an apothecary,' Otto asked with a polite smile.

'Not bloody likely. I'm a solicitor. Some fool I hired is running my practice while I sit here and listen to this drivel. I'm Town Clerk, sir.' Doctor Volkmann nodded at Otto Schaefer, then turned to face Rhinehart. 'You heard Clarus say that the university will never move against new ideas and freedom of speech. He knows damn well they can't. Just more hot air, like I'm hearing here.'

'Why not move a motion that we refuse to fill any prescriptions supplied by a homeopath,' Rhinehart responded angrily.

'Now you are losing your mind, Rhinehart,' cried the tall, blond man at the back. 'That would just open up the door for them to start dispensing their own medicines. Open up that precedent and you might as well say goodbye to your pension.'

'He's right,' added Volkmann. 'You might even get into trouble with the city's fathers for restraint of trade.'

'Gentlemen, gentlemen, do we have a motion or not?' asked the chairman. 'Time is fast escaping us.'

'At least we should agree to keep an eye on them,' Albert

Wagner said, climbing to his feet. 'I see the sense of what Doctor Volkmann is saying but we need to agree as a group that our livelihoods are potentially threatened unless we can in some way keep these homeopaths under control.'

'I agree,' one man shouted.

'Hear, hear,' came another cry from the back of the room.

'Then get on with it,' came a call from the far side, 'give us your motion. My stomach is telling me that something else is more important than these bloody homeopaths.'

A snigger ran like a wave through the room, even Albert Wagner had a smile on his face.

'I suggest we put a motion forward that ensures this group remains vigilant,' Wagner said, 'and which gives us the capacity to respond if something were to occur that threatens our income.'

'And how would you phrase such a motion, Herr Wagner?' asked Beck.

'Lets say that the apothecaries of Leipzig are watching ... no, no. The Leipzig apothecaries hereby agree that although the current status of homeopathy and of its practicing physicians should be tolerated, any change in the current circumstances will be viewed as a potential threat to the well-being of the apothecaries of this city and challenged forthwith.'

'Did you get all that, Beck?' Rhinehart shouted.

Frantically the chairman scribbled out the words, mumbling to himself as the quill sped across the paper. 'Right, I think I have it all.' He looked up from the paper in his hand. 'Did everyone understand the motion as put forward by Herr Wagner?'

A murmur of assent spread through the room.

'Is there anyone, then, who will second the motion?'

'I will,' cried Rhinehart. 'I'll second it and, in doing so, I promise everyone of you that I'll be watching these men very closely, very closely indeed.'

Albert Wagner nodded his head, steely determination blazing from his eyes, his fists clenched so tight that his skin showed white at the knuckles.

43

Otto Schaefer banged impatiently on Samuel's door. He halted for a brief moment then banged again. After a while it swung open. Caroline stood in the doorway, her pretty face flushed, her breathing slightly ragged. 'Herr Schaefer, I feared that the French must have returned.'

'My apologies, Fraulein. I very much wanted to talk to your father before the others joined him.'

'I'm afraid Karl has beaten you,' she smiled mischievously, 'although it would not require too much persuasion to keep him in the kitchen a little longer.'

Otto smiled as he walked into the house. 'Would it be too much of a burden? I really would value five minutes alone with your father.'

'I would be surprised if Franz and Ernst will arrive for at least another fifteen minutes. Would that be sufficient time?'

Caroline stopped at the door to her father's study and knocked. 'Father?' she smiled at the apothecary. 'Father, Herr Schaefer has arrived.'

A muffled noise came from inside the room. Caroline leant forward and opened the door.

'Otto, come in, come in. Thank you, Caroline. Have any of the others arrived yet?' Samuel climbed to his feet, his hand outstretched.

'Only Karl Franz, and he is in the kitchen enjoying a cup of tea with mama and I. I will bring him in when the others get here.' Without waiting for her father to reply, Caroline winked at Otto Schaefer and closed the study door behind her.

'I'm sorry to arrive early, Samuel, but I have been biting my tongue all afternoon waiting for your surgery to finish.'

'I thought you had a meeting with your fellow apothecaries this morning, Otto. Didn't that keep you busy?'

'Busy is hardly the word I would use to describe it,' he replied, poker-faced. 'The meeting ended around midday and I chose not to join any of them for lunch. So I have been forced to constrain myself until now.'

'Constrain yourself from what, my dear fellow?' Samuel asked with a broad smile.

'Samuel, you must never tell anyone where you heard what I am just about to tell you.'

'Otto, you are not making much sense. What have you heard that requires you to swear me to secrecy?'

'It is both what I have heard and who I heard it from. It appears to have escaped your notice, Samuel, that I am an apothecary. I make my living from dispensing medicines.'

'How can I forget it? I trust you implicitly, but I feel guilty when I force you to share our discoveries and our evolution, knowing that it goes against the grain of probably everything you were taught at business school.'

'You mean pharmacy school, Samuel,' Otto said, a perplexed look on his face.

'No, I meant exactly what I said.' Samuel's eyes sparkled with mischief. 'I am convinced that you apothecaries study the principles of business for years before you finally study any of the disciplines of medicine.'

'You mock me when I have some truly fascinating news to impart.' Otto's expression assumed a serious look. 'I spoke briefly with Doctor Stapf this morning and mentioned that I was attending the apothecary's meeting. At the time I facetiously said that I could not see how the meeting could reach a conclusion

without some reference to you and homeopathy.'
'And did your flippant remark prove accurate?'
'It certainly did.'
'Well then you are right, it does sound interesting.'
'Yes, it is, but it also leaves me in something of a quandary.'
'How so?'
'Even though I don't necessarily agree with everything my colleagues do or say, at the heart of it I am still one of them, and I'm still loyal to my roots.'
'I respect that, Otto. As I said before, I trust you. I had hoped that you would have the same confidence about me and would need no such reassurance.'

For the next ten minutes Otto described what had taken place at the society's meeting. He gave a fair account of the main antagonists and those he saw as potential allies, and launched a scathing attack on the chairman. When the story reached the treachery of Clarus and Dzondi, Samuel snorted and refused to be drawn. Otto finished his account with a question.
'What is your impression of Doctor Volkmann?'
'I think he is fair and honourable. Since the typhus business I have only seen him twice, both times at the university when we have attended the same function. My work doesn't usually bring me into contact with the city's administrators.' Samuel scratched his bald pate. 'I think I may have put him offside when I dredged up some of my old precepts of sanitation and the sorry state of our streets.' Otto's brow creased but Samuel waved the silent query aside. 'Remind me at another time, it is just another of the many ways I seem to have of annoying people.'
'So you have never had any reason to discuss homeopathy with him?'
'Briefly, after the typhus outbreak. He expressed gratitude on behalf of the city for the work I had done.'
'Well then, clearly he has done some homework on you. He gave the impression that he understood the concepts.'
'Perhaps an avid reader? I've certainly been copious in that

direction,' he smiled. 'Should I read into your question that you see Volkmann as a friend?'

'Absolutely. He made it clear that he would not suffer fools and, frankly, the meeting had its fair share of those.' Otto ran a hand over his heavy jowls while pondering his next comment. 'In the end, the motion passed at the meeting was so innocuous as to be almost a waste of the time getting to it. But the fact that the meeting was held at all should ring alarm bells in your head.'

'Oh, it does ...' Samuel began.

Otto was not quite finished. 'Given the chance, some of these men will be like a dog at a bone. They will keep at it until a weakness emerges, then they will pick the very marrow from it. Schaefer again stroked his jowls, deep in contemplation. 'But first they must find the weakness and, I suspect, that will only arise if you give them one.'

'Young Karl will no doubt become one of this country's greatest botanists if he doesn't become one of our best homeopaths,' Samuel said as Otto shook Karl Franz's hand.

'My other young colleagues also bring with them a passion for our trade, as well as their own speciality. Ernst,' Samuel nodded to the young Baron, who was reclining in one of the chairs in Samuel's study, 'has become our scribe. But that is far too clinical a description. He brings our meanderings and pontifications to life. I am also hugely respectful of him for he speaks French with the most beautifully fluent tongue. He has threatened one day to translate the *Organon* into French. If anyone ever succeeds in that it will advance homeopathy more so than any of my pathetic struggles here in Leipzig.'

'As usual, our good doctor maligns himself,' Franz Hartmann whispered into Otto's ear. The young student had remained standing beside the apothecary during the introductions.

'What was that? What did he say, Otto?' Samuel blustered good-naturedly.

'He said you need to see an apothecary to get some drugs for your hearing.' Otto turned to Franz Hartmann. 'Or did you say humility?'

'I should have known it would be dangerous to put you two together. Our young friend is far too open to ideas besides homeopathy,' Samuel replied, smiling.

'I thought I heard you commend Franz for that same attribute last night. Or perhaps I should also pay a visit to one of my colleagues for these hearing pills that Herr Hartmann is promoting.'

'Something tells me that neither of you should desert your chosen professions; the beer halls and theatres have comics aplenty.' Samuel clapped his hands. 'Enough! Otto, I promised to show you how we go about our provings. In doing so I can only hope that you will observe our earnestness and our diligence, and spread the word amongst your colleagues. Like everything in this world, ignorance is the enemy. The more people who understand what we do and why, the more likely it is that we will gain converts.'

'You have my wholehearted support on that. This morning's meeting is adequate testimony to the problem of ignorance,' Otto replied, noting the raised eyebrows and questioning looks on the faces of the three young men. 'I attended ...' Otto began to explain before catching the cautioning eye of Samuel Hahnemann. With an almost imperceptible nod he continued. 'I attended a meeting of some of my colleagues this morning and it is disappointing to hear some of their comments about something they don't truly understand.'

'Or more to the point, don't want to understand,' interjected von Brunnow. 'We are grateful, Herr Schaefer, that there are clearly some enlightened men amongst your group. However, as Doctor Hahnemann says, it is our responsibility to ensure more people come to understand, which is why I offered my skills as a writer, raw as they are.'

'How many are there in your group of collaborators now, Samuel?' Otto asked.

'At the moment: fourteen — thirteen who actually undertake the proving and the Baron who diligently writes up our ramblings and turns them into prose.'

'Obviously not all are yet qualified.'

'No. There's Stapf, of course, but mostly they are students and my own family.'

'Which begs the question, Samuel, how you ensure the credibility of your provings against the cynicism of my colleagues and the doctors?'

'The answer is simple, although painstaking,' Samuel replied. 'Each time my colleagues or my family and friends deliver their written records on provings, I question them in exhaustive detail to ensure that their verbal recollections are consistent with their recorded words.'

'Stapf talked about diet and even restrictions on activities,' Otto prompted.

Samuel nodded. 'Absolutely critical, but I don't check that they have complied with those rules. I don't need to. The discipline of proving is well understood by the group. If anyone should deviate it would be for a particular reason, and they would tell me. I don't have to hound them.'

'Each of us is committed to the procedures becoming so refined that they become a science in their own right, Herr Schaefer,' Karl Franz said from his chair.

'That's right,' interjected Franz Hartmann, 'I for one would not be subjecting my body or my health if I did not believe that, ultimately, this work will be recognised as a critical part of the practice of medicine.'

'Gentlemen, that is all well and good, but surely the flaw in the system is that everything has to come back through Samuel. He has to vet everything that is done.'

'Surely that is the nature of anything new in science,' Samuel pointed out. 'There has to be a pioneer, and if I have to wear that pithy title, so be it. But Stapf is already conducting his own provings without my weight at his shoulder. How else could he stay involved given the distance between us. For three years, Johann followed my instructions to the letter and recorded everything. Today there is no-one at the university who would dare refute our process, or that Stapf is not as accurate as I in his observations.'

'Once I have obtained my degree and am in practice, I will continue to undertake provings,' Franz Hartmann added. 'Who knows, within a decade there might be thirty of us working shoulder to shoulder proving the efficacy of medicines. Wouldn't that be a wonder to behold?'

'Herr Schaefer, what worries me,' Karl Franz interjected, 'is not whether we can support the premise of our provings, but whether people such as your colleagues will ever acknowledge their prejudices and embrace a system that delivers health to people rather than profit to apothecaries and doctors. And I say that with the greatest respect to your own position, sir, because I know it must be a difficult one. Yet I cannot help but think that homeopathy does not represent a sufficiently large money chest to the apothecaries, and for that reason alone they will never embrace it.'

Otto looked puzzled. 'I have heard my colleagues talk of the complexities of dispensing your products. I believe I understand the principle of dispensing that you adhere to, but my reason for maintaining a friendship,' Otto Schaefer smiled at Samuel, 'is because of our philosophical concurrence rather than anything practical. Frankly, I couldn't give a damn if the medicine you dispensed was no more than a thimble full, I would still fight for your right to cure people.'

'Well said, Herr Schaefer,' Franz Hartmann applauded, 'but most times it is not even a thimble full.'

'I was speaking metaphorically, sir.'

'And I am speaking literally,' replied Hartmann. 'Perhaps, Herr Schaefer, you would permit me to explain what is probably one of the most contentious principles of homeopathy.'

'I would be grateful for the lesson, young man.'

'I recall you saying last night that you had read the *Organon*,' Hartmann said.

Otto nodded.

'Unfortunately very little about the dosage question

appeared in the first edition, and a great deal has happened since then. 'Of particular interest is the work done by Doctor Hahnemann in determining dosage size, and the fact that we are starting to prove that the greater the dilution of a medicine, the more effective it can become.'

'What amount of dilution are you talking about?'

'As much as one fifty thousandth of a grain.'

'One fifty thous...!' Otto exploded. 'How in heaven's name can anyone measure one fifty thousandth of a grain and then correctly administer it?'

'Franz is being a little extreme, Otto,' Samuel interjected. 'For the moment I would only recommend that potency in ferrum. Something like arsenicum ...'

Otto laughed, 'How can you call something that small as potent?'

'David proved you don't have to be big to be potent, Otto,' Samuel rejoined.

'Look, I understand the principles, I truly do,' Otto Schaefer said, 'but you can't be serious. I would brush twenty times, no, a hundred times that amount of ferrum off my counter each I time I prepare a medicine with it.'

'Which is one of the issues that people like Clarus are using to fire up your colleagues and the doctors in town,' Hartmann added.

Otto waved Hartmann's interruption aside. 'How on earth do you measure such minuscule amounts, Samuel?'

'By dilution, of course; usually in a mixture of alcohol and water, no differently than you do, Otto.'

'What do you mean, no differently than I do?' Otto asked incredulously. 'I have never diluted anything to fifty thousandth of a single grain.'

'Otto, calm down, how can we persuade anyone if even you find it incredulous?' Samuel took his friend's arm and walked across to a table set up against the wall. Bottles and small phials of liquid were arranged across the surface.

'This really is no different to your first chemistry class at business school, Otto,' Samuel said with a cheeky grin that earned a scowl from the apothecary. 'The number of dilutions determines the potency.' Samuel picked up a piece of chalk and scrawled a 1 followed by an x on a small blackboard. 'The first centesimal potency, or 1x, consists of one part of the mother tincture and nine parts of an alcohol water base.' Samuel reached in front of Otto and picked up a small phial no larger than two inches high and half an inch wide. A small stopper had been inserted into the mouth of the slim tube that was three quarters filled with a clear fluid. 'This already contains a measure of the first centesimal. If I add one part of this mixture to a further nine of the alcohol-water mixture then I achieve my second potency, or 2x.' Again Samuel scrawled the number and letter on the blackboard. He put the chalk down and picked up a second phial. 'The third potency is achieved by adding one part of this second phial to another containing nine parts of the alcohol-water mix. And so on. As I said, it really is no different to your own methods.'

'I can understand that, Samuel, and I'm also beginning to understand how Clarus and his cronies, not to mention my own colleagues, are trying to whip this up into a storm. What you are describing is a very complex and time-consuming process.'

'It doesn't need to be, Otto, if the various potencies of each remedy are kept, already prepared.'

'Samuel, how many apothecaries can you see doing that? My goodness, no wonder there is a bellyache developing.'

'So you see part of our dilemma?'

Otto nodded, stroking his jowls pensively.

'And what are you thinking, my dear friend?'

'Eh?' Otto replied, distractedly.

'Whenever you start to pull at your cheeks, I know something is going on in that brain of yours.'

Otto nodded. 'Maybe I was a trifle hasty, perhaps there is a way to make this work for all parties.' Otto scratched his belly. 'If the apothecaries didn't want to keep all of the remedies required then the apothecary could sell the homeopath a licence to make and dispense their own on condition that the homeopath purchase their primary ingredients from the local apothecary. Look sir, I don't know if that is a practical solution, but something could be worked out of a similar nature. What is important is that everyone understands why.'

'But there would be very little profit in it for the pharmacist,' argued Franz Hartmann.

'Then the pharmacist would need to expand his options, consider where else he could apply the principles of trade. What we are really debating here is the need to accept change, if we are to ensure we put the health of our public first.' Otto added. 'All that aside, I'm more concerned about how you persuade the world that something that can not be seen under a microscope is anything more than a placebo. David may have slain Goliath with a sling, but from all the reports I've read, he was still a fairly strapping lad.'

44

'I am reminded of a recent conversation with a learned friend who found it difficult to understand the concept of potency as achieved through dilution and dynamisation.'

Samuel Hahnemann stood at the front of his class, a copy of the new edition of the *Organon* in his hand. Unconsciously he rubbed his fingers over the raised gold print on the cover.

Attendances had fallen since the first year, but today word had spread that the professor would be unveiling a new edition of his life work, his first book in nearly four years. Several members of the faculty, attempting to hide at the back of the room, had joined the swollen student numbers. They were the first faces Samuel saw when he made his entrance. He laughed quietly to himself at their attempted subterfuge.

'In the first edition,' Samuel continued, holding the book aloft, 'I spent little time discussing the dosage, concentrating perhaps too much on the philosophical side of things. In part that is why my friend's timely reminder caused me to revisit the subject today. Perhaps one of the younger students would indulge me with an explanation of what he understands the term "succussing" to mean?'

Samuel looked around. Young Hartmann sat with his good friend, Hornburg, in the front row. Deliberately Samuel ignored the two collaborators, his eyes scanning the rest of the room.

Finally a hand was tentatively poked into the air. Samuel recognised the hirsute young man from his last lecture, his bristling beard reminding him of one of his other students, who was also one of the collaborators. This was only the second time that Samuel had seen him in attendance.

'Yes, young sir, you in the second row. I apologise, but your name has escaped me for the moment,' Samuel said with a self-conscious smile.

'Rückert, Doctor Hahnemann, Theodor Rückert, my brother Ernst is already known to you,' the young man replied, his eyes sparkling above the dense black of his beard.

'Herr Rückert,' Samuel nodded, 'please enlighten us.'

'The term "succuss" means to shake or shake up. Homeopathically, it refers to the action of mixing the proposed remedy by vigorously shaking the mixture in its container.'

'Thank you, Herr Rückert, that is exactly what it means. Would you be prepared to expand your explanation as to the importance of succussing the remedy?' Samuel asked.

'It would be an honour,' Rückert replied. 'I believe it starts with your own stated intention: to attain the ideal cure — one that is rapid, gentle, permanent and reliable.'

Samuel raised his eyebrows in surprise.

'There is a good body of evidence that clearly shows homeopathic treatment can now achieve cures that are perhaps more rapid and reliable than allopathic remedies. However ... forgive me if my reply is outside the specific intent of your question.'

'I am fascinated with your approach. Please continue,' Samuel replied with an encouraging smile.

'Well, what I intended to say,' the youngster continued nervously, 'is that perhaps the remedies weren't quite as gentle as you would have liked.'

'Damned right, young man!' Samuel cried, nodding his head vigorously. 'They were almost pure poison, but they worked.'

A gentle ripple of chuckles rose from the audience and then died behind raised hands.

Rückert tried to hide his own smile, his confidence growing in the shadow of the master's display of eccentricity. 'Quite. And they were tolerated by patients who were already accustomed to being bled or given toxic doses of mercury and opiates.'

A roar of laughter engulfed the theatre, the students unable to contain themselves any longer. At the back of the room the two members of the faculty began to rise in unison and then thought better of it, dropping back into their seats before they were noticed.

'You will have to excuse your fellows, Herr Rückert,' Samuel said directly to the young student, a twinkle in his eyes. 'I can assure you that they are laughing at me not at your good self. Perhaps they are also laughing at their own inadequacy to answer the question as intelligently as you are doing. Please continue.'

'Er, thank you, Doctor Hahnemann,' Rückert replied, a faint blush rising above the beard. 'Well, I was going to add that your efforts at diluting the remedies were not always successful.'

Samuel shook his head, mumbling, 'On that point you are most assuredly right.'

'Sorry, Doctor Hahnemann, I didn't catch your comment,' Franz Hartmann interjected from his place at the front.

'I said, Herr Hartmann, that Herr Rückert is correct. I tried many different potencies, as you well know.' Samuel finished with a steely look in his eye. He turned to Rückert, well aware of Hartmann's surreptitious wink to Hornburg. 'Herr Rückert, please excuse these rude interruptions and continue.'

'Thank you, doctor. What I had intended to say was that, although not always successful, ultimately your trial and error led you to the conclusion that simply by diluting the remedies they would eventually have no effect, which is when you turned to the idea of thoroughly mixing each remedy by succussing it.'

'And not only did it work,' Samuel exclaimed to the lecture room, 'once succussed they appeared to have more potency and more curative power than the most concentrated dosages.' Samuel beamed out over his audience before remembering himself. He looked at his new student. 'I am very impressed at your grasp, sir. I can only assume that your brother has been a very good tutor or that you have managed to find yourself a copy of the new edition.' Again Samuel held up the heavy volume. 'Much of what you have said is still new, even to those who have been attending these lectures for some years.' Samuel nodded to Rückert who basked in the glory of Samuel's praise.

'Succussing the remedy,' Samuel continued, 'is part of what I have come to call "potentisation". Those of you working with me on the proving of medicines will already be familiar with the term. For the rest of you, I suspect it sounds more like something our very own Goethe may have written about in one of his science fantasies.' A nervous tinkle of laughter came from the newer students. Samuel smiled at his sally before continuing. 'I said at the commencement that today's lecture was prompted by a colleague, a friend who found it hard to accept that something diluted until it contained no more than a fifty thousandth of a grain...'

'What!' The strangled cry came from the back of the room. Almost as one, the student's turned just as the member of faculty clamped a hand to his mouth.

'So, Doctor Karl, you also find that a little difficult to comprehend? Then perhaps you should close your ears to what I am to say next. Although I have no proof, not substantive proof anyway, I am convinced that even if we dilute the remedy to a point where there is not a single molecule of the original substance remaining, the remedy will still have the power to cure the patient.'

A loud exhalation of air cut through the room.

'This is preposterous ...' Doctor Karl had risen to his feet at the back of the room. Slowly his colleague joined him, the two men standing with mouths agape.

'Oh, for goodness sake, Karl, either sit down and let us get on with the lecture or leave. At the moment both of you look like fish gasping for air out of water.'

'Hahnemann, this time I swear you have gone too far,' Karl

shouted as he fled the room, his colleague stumbling along behind.

Samuel waited as the noise in the room abated and then, with a broad smile, held his hands in the air. 'Gentlemen, now that our spies have departed I am sure there are some of you who may feel inclined to join them, suspecting that I truly have gone mad. Let me assure you, nothing could be further from the truth.' Samuel looked at each student in the room. No-one made a move.

When he was sure of their attention he continued. 'In 1811, Avogadro published an article in *Journal de Physique* that clearly drew the distinction between the molecule and the atom. In it he pointed out that not only had Dalton confused the concepts of atoms and molecules but he had also hypothesised that, through dilution, there is a measurable point where not a single molecule of substance remains.' Again Samuel paused, his hands on his hips. 'Now what has that to do with my assertion?' He looked around the room waiting for a response, his broad smile still in place. 'Nobody wants to comment?' he asked. 'Well, thank goodness for that because it has nothing to do with anything. I just didn't want any of you to think that I didn't understand my chemistry.'

A huge roar of laughter rose from the seated students.

Samuel held up his hands. 'Please, it is time to become serious once more. The ancient Greeks have a name for what I want to discuss. They call it dynamis. Others have called it the vital force, and I choose to call it the life principle.' Samuel carefully studied the reactions of the students before continuing. 'In essence I am suggesting that the effects of our homeopathic remedies have nothing to do with biochemistry at all, or at least do not act on the material body alone. I suspect that when diluted to the maximum potency our remedies act on an entirely energised or non-physical plane.'

'Doctor Hahnemann.'

Samuel turned to face the young man waiting outside the lecture room. He recognised Professor Ludwig's earnest secretary, his lanky frame constantly bowed from deferring to the academia around him.

'Herr Schmidt, to what do I owe this pleasure?' Samuel asked, a polite smile fixed to his face.

Schmidt bobbed his head repeatedly, anxiously wringing his hands. 'Professor Ludwig has asked if you would attend him in his rooms. Apparently there is an important matter he wishes to discuss with you.'

'An important matter? What could be more important than returning to spend what remains of my Saturday with my family?' Samuel cocked an eyebrow.

'Er, well, Doctor Hahnemann, I'm not rightly sure. Just that the Professor insisted that it was important. He, um, invited Professor Clarus to join him, but he, er, asked me not to tell you that, sir.'

Perversely Samuel pulled out his fob watch in a display of impatience and then turned on his heel. 'Come on then, Schmidt. Let's get this disciplinary hearing over and done with.

Ludwig paced the floor in front of the fireplace, his hands washing nervously behind his back. Clarus sat in the armchair opposite Samuel, his legs stretched out in front of him, a cold glare in his eyes and a thin smile on his lips. Ludwig stopped his pacing and turned to Samuel.

'Doctor, I must insist.' The Dean switched his hands from behind his back, but continued washing them in front of his two visitors. 'The university has given you a mandate to deliver lectures to our students — on medicine, sir, not on fantasy.'

Samuel had his eyes fixed on Clarus as the Dean continued his tirade. Clarus had not said a word.

'As if none of this were enough, we have this ridiculous mud slinging in the press between you and Dzondi. Mud slinging that is splattering its dirt all over the university, sir!'

'I must agree,' Clarus cut in, his words cold and biting. Out of the corner of his eye Samuel saw the Dean heave a sigh of relief at the interruption.

'This so-called dispute has been raging for over a year now, Doctor Hahnemann,' Clarus continued. His eyes bored into Samuel's. 'The medical world is well aware of your role here at the university so no matter how much you bluster and protest to the contrary, what you say in the press and the journals has the potential for serious backlash on the university.'

Seated at his desk, Dean Ludwig was nodding his head, hanging on to each word. Samuel remained strangely calm, waiting for the right moment to make his attack.

'If I am correct, Doctor Hahnemann, you were granted your position here at the university thanks to your dissertation on white hellebore, in which, again if my memory serves, you spoke very much from the provinces of medical history. In fact I will go one step further and suggest that not once during your dissertation did you allude to any of your pet theories or so-called principles.'

Clarus paused to take breath, his eyes still locked on Samuel's. 'For more than three years we have tolerated you spreading your principles, and have watched as some of the university's brightest students have been cast under your spell. Now we have this farcical business with Professor Dzondi, who wisely preaches *contraria contraries* — something every one of your university colleagues is comfortable with, I should add.' Finally the professor's demeanour cracked, the glacial tones replaced by an imperious sneer that resonated through his voice. 'Yet not only do you persist with your contradictions, you now seem determined to take all of us into the realms of fantasy.

'So what are we to take from all of this?' the university's Clinical Professor continued belligerently, 'That you hold your position here under false pretences?' The professor glared at Samuel, and then shook his head. 'I'm not sure which is the greater crime — that you have duped us from the very beginning into believing you would follow a conservative path in the lecturing of medicine, or this latest insult, where you appear determined to turn your lectures into something that would be more befitting a literature class. Perhaps we should assume the role of referees and make a personal representation on your behalf to Goethe. He and his literary fellows would no doubt enjoy your trips into fantasy.'

Samuel's knuckles were white, the line of his mouth thin. Slowly he exhaled, releasing the anger that coursed through him. 'Have I the right of reply, Dean Ludwig?' Samuel's eyes continued to bore into Clarus, the glare returned with an equally fierce determination not to cede ground.

'Well, er ... I, of course you do ... Doctor Hahnemann,' Ludwig blustered.

'Thank you.' Samuel said. 'Professor Clarus, when a chef burns his hand he never uses cold water but holds his hand close to the burning coals until the pain has diminished to the point where it is almost gone. In so doing he knows that there will be no water blister and that the injury will resolve itself in a short space of time without any subsequent pain. If you don't believe me, go and ask the chef at your favourite eating-house. Likewise, the experience of daily life, sir, is filled with examples of *similia similibus*. The famed British surgeon, Benjamin Bell, who I understand you are an outspoken champion for, has publicly supported this very same treatment for burns. As has Heister and others.' Samuel held Clarus with his eyes.

'My dissertation was deliberately written to draw everyone's attention to the problem that my students and I are painstakingly undertaking to resolve.' Samuel paused a moment to allow the thought to settle. 'I was actually applauded at the conclusion of my address, professor, as you no doubt remember.' He inclined his head towards the Dean, not once taking his eyes from Clarus. 'Am I not correct, Dean Ludwig? If I recall, you added your own voice to the congratulations.

'Yes, yes, I did. But I'm not sure I clearly understand your comment about you and your students, Doctor Hahnemann.'

'White hellebore or, as we would know it, veratrum album, is one of hundreds of medicines that can be traced back to the ancients. It has been used to treat people for centuries and yet no-one has ever clinically proven exactly what it does, or why.

Of course we know that it has been successful in treating the symptoms for which it has been prescribed, but in truth the proof is no better than anecdotal. Have there ever been tests to show what other effects the medicine might be having on the body of the patient or whether it has contributed to other conditions?' Samuel shook his head. 'Regrettably the answer is no, there have not.

'With only the smallest number of exceptions, most of the medicines written up in the volumes of medical tomes have been discovered purely by chance. I can count the exceptions on one hand.' Samuel ticked his fingers. 'Perhaps marsh fever and venereal diseases, and of course cloth-worker's itch. To this we could add the accidental discovery of preservation from smallpox by vaccination. How ironic is it, that these three or four cures are all effected through the principle of *similia similibus*? Since the time of Hippocrates, the cure of all other diseases has remained unknown.'

'This is preposterous!' Clarus exclaimed, half rising in his seat.

'I thought I had the right of reply, Dean Ludwig, or do the clinicians now hold sway over academia?'

'No, of course not ... please Professor Clarus,' Ludwig appealed to his colleague. 'But, like Professor Clarus, I would welcome you making your point, sir, and quickly.'

Clarus dropped back into his seat, hate simmering behind his eyes.

'You, gentlemen, have dragged me in here on the pretext that I am spreading fantasy and preaching fairy stories.'

Clarus exploded. 'What else should we think when you suggest that a phial of water or water mixed with alcohol and nothing else could cure someone of anything.'

'Professor, please,' pleaded Ludwig.

'If your spies had not been so intent on cutting and running,' Samuel interrupted, 'they would have learned that I was not suggesting that at all.

What I was about to say when they so abruptly left was

nothing more nor less than an extension of the principles propounded by Stahl, or those of Hippocrates himself, or even the theories of the French vitalists. All of them talked about the soul or the *force vitale*, the life power that is invisible to any doctor, allopathic or homeopathic. That is where I was leading when your lackeys suddenly felt so intimidated.'

'Don't treat me like a fool,' Clarus stormed, not even bothering to hide his exclusion of the Dean. 'You think you can fool your young students with your silver tongue, Hahnemann, but you do not deceive me. Karl and Franks both clearly heard you talk about witchcraft.'

'What I said had nothing to do with witchcraft and was clearly taken out of context. My comments were a legitimate hypothesis.' Samuel paused and turned to Ludwig. 'Is it still the university's position to foster new thinking, Dean?' Without waiting for a response Samuel returned his attention to Clarus. 'A principle I understand you protected to the hilt at a recent meeting of apothecaries.'

'What? Where did you hear ...?'

'My dear sir, you should never underestimate the homeopathic network. I made the remark that even if we were to dilute the homeopathic remedy to a point where there is not a single molecule of the original substance left, that it will still have the power to cure the patient if we have followed the process correctly and accurately.'

'And you don't call that witchcraft, sir?'

'I call it exploring new ideas, Professor Clarus,' Samuel responded calmly. 'You are either blind or illiterate, or even worse, ignorant, if you have not followed the development of life force concepts. For centuries theologians have believed that each of us has a soul. Fortunately, today I am not the only doctor to believe that a spirit-like life force helps the body function. I do not accept that bodily disease is completely physical, as you and your colleagues do. I will never just accept. More to the point, I am not convinced that anyone will ever completely understand how the body functions. Nor am I sure that it is necessary for us to do so to successfully practice medicine.'

'This is pure bunkum, Ludwig,' Clarus remarked with an imperious tone.

'Discovery is only bunkum to those not prepared to make the journey, Professor Clarus. And you and your colleagues are clearly too frightened to embark on a journey to the unknown. Your view of the body is mechanistic in the extreme. You believe that you can't repair what you can't see. But what if you can't completely know how something works? Do we then give up? Do we stop seeking the answers?' Samuel shook his head sadly. Slowly he climbed to his feet. 'Dean Ludwig, I can see no reason for us to continue this conversation. If the university intends to withdraw my commission then so be it. I will go elsewhere to continue my work.' Samuel then turned to face Professor Clarus. 'I believe that people are intrinsically self-healing and that what we doctors do is help facilitate that process. Historically we have focused on the treatment of a single symptom. I believe that to be wrong and I am determined to prove it.'

PART SIX

LEIPZIG, 1819-1821

45

'Herr Schaefer, what a delightful surprise. Papa made no comment that you were visiting.' Caroline held the front door open for Otto.

'Unfortunately I had little chance to send a message ahead of my travel.' Otto removed his hat and smiled distractedly at Samuel's daughter.

'I'm afraid that papa may be a little while, he has a rather busy schedule this morning.'

Otto looked over the young woman's shoulder into the waiting room. Nearly every seat was taken. A young mother with a small child waited patiently for Caroline to return to her duties.

'My apologies, Fraulein, I should have thought ... but I have some important news ...' Otto fiddled with his hat. 'How long do you think he will be?'

'The rest of the morning at least,' Caroline offered with a smile. 'Perhaps if you have no other business you might like to wait in the parlour. I'm sure you will be able to find something interesting to read besides medical volumes.'

Otto offered Caroline a tentative smile. 'Perhaps if your mother is at home I could presume on the delightful lady to share a cup of tea.'

'I'm sorry, mama is out. I don't expect her back before lunch at the earliest. She has even left instructions for Frederika to prepare our midday meal, which of course you are most welcome to join.'

'I don't wish to be a nuisance.' Otto thought about it then said, 'Thank you, yes, that would be admirable. I have no other business here today except to talk to your father.'

'Otto, how wonderful to see you. You are joining us for lunch?' Samuel Hahnemann crossed to the chair where Otto had made himself comfortable, a copy of the *Organon* in his lap. The two men shook hands warmly. 'So tell me, what news do you bring?'

'Well, first, an old friend of yours asked to be remembered to you,' Otto said. 'Name of Heinz. He runs a busy coach business in Dresden. Says you might remember him from your time in the mad house. Is this something I should know about Samuel?'

Samuel smiled fondly as he settled into a chair facing the apothecary. 'Heinz was my saviour on many occasions, including saving me from the madhouse. But no, you needn't worry about my sanity, now or at any time in the past.'

Otto smiled back. 'One day you will have to tell me the story.'

'It's a long time ago, before you and I met. But tell me, where did you come across Heinz, and how, for goodness sakes, did my name come up?'

'Well, he just so happens to be my new partner. And his son was the coachman who brought me here.'

'Your partner?' Samuel asked, surprised. 'And surely you mean his stepson. If I recall correctly his wife had only the one child and they had none between them.'

Otto shook his head, a broad smile on his face. 'Heinz and his wife now have a brood of four children. Nothing to compare to your own of course, as Heinz was quick to point out. You are obviously aware that he and his wife found it hard to have a family, then when she was approaching forty she discovered she was with child. Some months later they were the proud parents of healthy twins, a girl and a boy. Not more than a year after that they had another girl. That's when Heinz sought me out.' Otto smiled wickedly. 'He came to my pharmacy in Dresden and asked if there was anything that could protect his wife from him.'

A soft knock on the door interrupted them. Caroline poked her head into the room. 'Papa, mother has returned and has announced lunch. She insists that you hurry; she is sure that Herr Schaefer must be starving.'

Samuel smiled as he climbed from his chair. 'Perhaps you can tell me what you prescribed for the poor man after lunch,' he said. 'Over lunch you must enlighten me about this partnership you have got yourself into.'

'More pie, Herr Schaefer? Mama says you need to build up your strength,' Frederika said, her eyes twinkling.

'Yes, I will, thank you,' Otto replied, his own eyes shining brightly. 'It is truly a strength-giving pie. I think I should also have some more of that health-enriched cream that your mama is so famous for.'

'Otto, I swear,' Samuel interrupted, 'I have not been able to get one word from you during lunch. Your respect for the importance of food does you credit, but sometimes too much of a good thing... ' Samuel glanced at his friend's girth, leaving the sentence unfinished.

Otto patted his stomach contentedly. 'Impatient to hear about my new partner, eh, Samuel? No doubt you will also want to know why I would decide to diversify at this time of my life.' For the briefest moment Otto turned his twinkling eyes on his friend before returning his attention to the heaped bowl in front of him.

'Something of that nature, yes.'

'The first part is easy,' Otto mumbled through a mouthful of pie and cream. The portly apothecary wiped his chin. 'Heinz moved to Dresden several years ago. He had the chance to take over a small transport company that had a lucrative trade with Prague.' Otto paused to spoon a chunk of pie and cream into his mouth.

'You may recall that you introduced me to Heinz in Molschleben,' Otto resumed, his napkin again at work.

Samuel nodded vaguely. 'If you say I did. I seem to recall that Heinz was grateful to me for introducing him to several people.'

'Oh, he is most definitely grateful. The business he started so many years ago in Gotha has become a thriving transport network across southern Saxony and into the northern parts of Austria.'

'Thanks in no small part to his very astute wife, I suspect,' added Samuel.

Otto swallowed another portion of pie. 'Mmm, in fact it was her persuasive skills that got me involved.' Otto looked affectionately at the spoon in his hand. 'Heinz sought me out when I first moved to Dresden, offering to undertake any freight work I needed. A few months ago he came to see me to seek my knowledge of Leipzig. Once again he was considering expanding and had the opportunity to buy out a struggling firm.'

'Here in Leipzig?' Samuel asked.

Otto nodded. 'This time he also mentioned that he was keen to seek a partner to help finance the purchase.'

'And you took up his offer?' Samuel asked in surprise.

'Well ... yes. I had been thinking for some time of getting out of the pharmacy business.'

'Then I would lose the only friend I have in that sphere of the world,' Samuel said, his eyebrows raised in mock horror.

'I can see how that grieves you,' Otto said with a smile. 'Truth is, I have often thought about our conversations. It may surprise you to know that under this rather large facade there is a conscience.'

Samuel laid a hand gently on Otto's sleeve. 'I never doubted it.'

'That is the real reason why I came here so urgently today, and is something with which I have been struggling all morning.'

'What, your conscience?' Samuel asked in good humour.

'Indirectly.' Otto spooned the last of the pie into his mouth and sighed contentedly. 'When Johanna returns from the kitchen I must congratulate her on a pie made in Heaven.'

'Otto, stop being so obtuse.' Samuel narrowed his eyes. 'Or do I detect that your delaying tactics are rooted in something much deeper? I think we should move to my study where we will not interfere with the rest of the family.'

'It's a long story,' Otto said as he settled into the comfortable armchair in Samuel's study. A cloud had taken the twinkle from his eyes. Samuel sat behind his desk, absently playing with a quill.

'The success of our new venture,' Otto began, 'is that Heinz has the skills and knowledge of the transport business whilst I have a network of contacts and friends that, you may be surprised to know, contains very few apothecaries.'

Samuel remained silent, his eyes focused on the feathers that sprang from the stem of the quill.

'Many of my contacts are in hospitals and universities, and even publishers here in Leipzig. Each one of those groups represented a new business opportunity for Heinz, a sensible diversification of his trade which for years has been concentrated on general trade. From my base in Dresden, I was already building a network through Austria and the surrounding nations. My travels often took me to Vienna and north to Prague, where I made a number of important contacts such as the Chief Physician of the Prague General Infirmary.'

'Joseph Bischoff?'

'Yes, do you know him?'

'Not personally, but he is very highly regarded by his peers and carries a great deal of influence. I remember he once wrote an article that acknowledged some of the work I was doing. I recall he spoke of his approval for the proving of medicine.'

'And he still does,' said Otto, 'to a point.'

'What do you mean?'

'I met with Bischoff, on a recent trip to Prague, to persuade the hospital to give us the contract to haul their medical supplies.'

'And were you successful?' Samuel looked up from the quill.

Otto looked smug. 'We now have the contract to supply

much of their general trade from Saxony and the whole German Confederation. Once you gain a toehold in some of these government contracts, you can write your own ticket.'

'With some careful oiling of the wheels,' Samuel observed.

'I leave all the mechanical problems to Heinz.'

A hint of impatience touched Samuel's eyes. Otto nodded, acknowledging that it was time to come to the point. 'I had dinner with Bischoff, and we began talking about changes in medicine. After a few glasses, he asked me if I had ever met you. I hedged and said that I had met you many years before at Molschleben, and left it at that. After another few glasses he came back to his question, by which time we had solved the problems of the world.'

Samuel nodded, not wishing to interrupt his friend's story.

'Again he spoke of you and explained to me that he had written a work titled *Views on the Methods of Healing up to this Time and on the First Principles of Homeopathy*.'

'The title specifically mentions homeopathy?' Samuel asked in surprise.

'Most assuredly; I have seen the manuscript. In fact I have just delivered it to the publisher here in Leipzig.'

'You delivered it?'

'Of course; it was a promise that helped secure the contract.'

'And you know what this manuscript contains?'

'Bischoff acknowledges your contributions to medicine. He approves of your methods in proving and preparation, but he rejects out of hand your homeopathic principles, claiming that conventional methods offer a much greater benefit for mankind. When he told me, he became very vehement in his condemnation of you for your attacks on bloodletting.'

'He is not the first,' Samuel said, resignation in his voice.

'Nor will he be the last, Samuel.' Otto leant forward in his chair. 'There are angry noises coming from the apothecaries of Dresden, Samuel. They feel that their livelihoods are being threatened by your colleagues, who openly dispense their own medicines. It would appear from my conversation with Bischoff that the same is occurring in Prague. I have been back in Leipzig less than twenty-four hours and I can already feel the tension here.'

'So what do you expect me to do — go forth into battle?' Samuel smiled sadly at his friend. 'Battle against whom?'

'Samuel, I came to warn you ...'

'And your warning is respected, believe me. I must admit that such a direct attack takes me by surprise. For some time now we have been nurturing friends in important places. You remember Volkmann?' Samuel looked up to see Otto nodding. 'A year or so ago he came to see me as a patient. His ills are now cured and he is a firm believer. I have even had correspondence from von Sax asking me to visit Austria to treat Prince Karl of Schwarzenberg.'

'What is wrong with him?' Otto asked, astounded.

'Apparently he suffered a serious stroke and is not responding to his physician's treatment. Not that I'm surprised. No amount of blood-letting will solve that condition.'

'When are you going?' Otto asked.

'I'm not. I can't desert my patients, no matter how important the new one may be.'

'But this is exactly the sort of patronage you need. Schwarzenberg still wields enormous power. Sick or not, he is still cousin to our king.'

Samuel shrugged his shoulders. 'Unfortunately his recovery must remain in the hands of his physicians and, regrettably, that probably means he will not recover.'

'Samuel, I despair. You should travel to Austria immediately, treat him and then seek his support.'

Samuel Hahnemann looked sadly at his good friend. 'That is not my way and you know it. I am settled and content with my life. Homeopathy will survive because it works, not because I gain royal patronage for it.'

Sadly Otto shook his head. 'Beware, Samuel, I fear the lions are closing. If you do not heed the warnings they will rip you to shreds.'

46

Johann Stapf waited patiently in the forecourt of the university's medical school. Around him the stone walls of the buildings brought back fond memories of his own studies. Students hurried past with the same sense of controlled urgency he remembered from his own examinations. He pulled his coat tight to cut out the cold wind that sliced through the courtyard.

'Johann, I'm sorry I'm late.' Franz Hartmann came to halt at Stapf's side, his breathing rushed. He held out a hand. 'Oh, how I wish I were in your position, Johann. The red tape is far worse than any examinations. And if Clarus makes one more attack on homeopathy I swear I will beat him to death with a copy of the *Organon*.'

'Calm yourself,' Stapf said with a smile. 'We all have to endure the same rigours before we can be loosed on any unsuspecting patients. I also had to sit the bachelor's examination and my *rigorosum* before I was finally able to deliver my doctor's dissertation. It took me nearly two years from my bachelor's to the final paper. And you forget that I also had to endure the good professor's savage tongue.'

'Perhaps not quite the same, Johann; the faculty did not vilify you for your association with Doctor Hahnemann at every turn. I swear there are times when I feel that he has forsaken any defence of his principles.'

Stapf acknowledged the point. 'You stated your concerns on that matter very clearly in your correspondence, Franz. And I don't need to be at the university to gain the same feeling.'

'Then what are we to do? Since Bischoff's paper was published earlier this year ...'

'What we are to do,' Stapf interrupted, 'is to find a warm inn where we can get something edible for lunch and a quiet corner to talk.'

Stapf pushed the empty bowl away and leant back in his chair. Franz Hartmann was wiping the last of the thick soup from his own bowl with a crust of bread.

'So how does it feel to have qualified?'

'Relieved. That's truly the only word I can use. Nor could I have achieved it if I had stayed here.' Hartmann wiped the corner of his mouth with a napkin then threw it onto the table beside his bowl. 'Now it remains to be seen whether I will be allowed to submit for the *viva voce* here.'

'So that is why you were at the university today?' Stapf said.

'I had to give my application to the new Dean.'

'Ludwig has finally retired?'

'Yes, although I'm not sure whether that is to our advantage or not. He may not have always appeared to be on our side, but at least he was sympathetic. It still remains to be seen which way Rosenmüller will jump.'

'If Clarus is still pulling the strings ...'

'Please don't mention that name,' Hartmann said, a grim smile on his face. 'Several of the graduating students have already felt the lash of his tongue. He wears his position as Medical Councillor on his sleeve. No-one dares breathe without looking over their shoulder.'

'So why have you returned? You could have applied in Jena.'

'I only went to Jena to avoid the persecution of the faculty, just as I went to Berlin for a year to escape the other students' animosities against homeopathy.'

'Stirred up wonderfully by Clarus and his mob.' Stapf smiled grimly.

'That is what prompted me to write to you. It seems for some time that we have been increasingly bearing the brunt of the university's antagonism towards homeopathy.'

'By "we", I assume you mean the students?' Stapf asked.

'Well, yes. The students and, of course, qualified physicians such as yourself. On the other hand, Doctor Hahnemann seems preoccupied with his practice, which increases in size every day.'

'Perhaps Samuel believes that the best way to spread the word is through his success with his patients. It appears to be working. My own practice is also thriving as the people of Naumberg realise that our cures are effective.'

'Then who is there to refute some of the attacks that are being levelled through the journals? I was in Jena when Bischoff's paper was published, yet I saw nothing to refute it. Doctor Hahnemann made no attempt to repel the criticisms Bischoff made.'

'Perhaps you should have taken up the quill and penned a response,' Stapf said quietly.

'And put my graduation at risk?' Hartmann cried.

'Quite,' said Stapf deliberately. He paused to look Hartmann in the eye. 'I have not spoken to Samuel for some time. However, I have become concerned at the growing unrest of the apothecaries in Naumberg. I received a delegation a few weeks ago; the message to desist from dispensing my own medicines was none too subtle. Your letter galvanised me to take a few days to come and visit with the good doctor. Perhaps we should visit him together and express our concerns.'

Hartmann sighed with relief. 'Thank you. I am sure Doctor Hahnemann will pay more attention to the warning if it comes from you rather than some of the younger provers.' The young man stopped and reached inside the satchel that lay on the floor at his feet. He pulled out a folded copy of Hufeland's journal and laid it on the table between them. 'Particularly now that Puchelt has joined in the attack.'

'Puchelt? What do you mean ...?' Stapf reached for the publication. 'Puchelt has always defended Samuel. What is he saying?'

'He flags the growth of homeopathy amongst younger doctors and the public.'

'So why should that concern you?'

'He uses it as a springboard to launch a scathing personal attack on Doctor Hahnemann, criticising the doctor for his disrespect for the medical science of healing.'

'No-one could deny that. Samuel has been its most vocal critic; he couldn't expect to maintain his attacks without someone coming out and returning fire.' Stapf turned his attention to the paper on the table. 'Do you think you are being completely fair, Franz?' Stapf pointed his finger at a paragraph half way down the page he was reading. 'Here, Professor Puchelt acknowledges that he will introduce homeopathy into his own teachings where it addresses dynamic troubles. Isn't that part of what we have been fighting for?'

Franz Hartmann nodded. 'There are parts, I agree, where Puchelt is sensitive to the principles of homeopathy.' Hartmann ran a hand through his thick hair. 'I suspect my anger is as much about the accuracy of Puchelt's comments, it is about the attack he raises.'

'You mean his comments about Doctor Hahnemann personally, rather than his principles.'

'Yes,' Hartmann said. 'At one point Puchelt opines that if Doctor Hahnemann had not declared open war on the rest of medicine then his theories might well now be part of the tradition.'

'Unfortunately the good professor may well have a point.'

Stapf closed the copy of the journal and sat staring at the cover. He looked up to see Hartmann watching him.

'Do you think Samuel has seen this?' Stapf asked.

'I doubt it.' Hartmann pointed to the magazine. 'I collected that copy only this morning, the ink is still wet from the presses. I also doubt whether Doctor Hahnemann is bothering to take the time to keep up with the popular press. He is so taken up with his practice that the world could be ending and he wouldn't know it.'

'Then I think it is our duty to appraise him of the facts,' Doctor Stapf said, rising to his feet.

47

'Doctor Volkmann? How are you ...?' Johann Stapf jumped to one side as the large frame of the Town Clerk slammed the door to Doctor Hahnemann's rooms and flew down the steps.

'Stapf?' Doctor Volkmann mumbled in surprise, stopping abruptly. 'Sorry, my dear fellow, I didn't see you there.' The Town Clerk peered at Franz. 'Hartmann isn't it?' I haven't seen either of you around for a while.'

'This is the first chance ...' Stapf began.

'God damn, Hahnemann,' Volkmann exploded, cutting Stapf off. 'Why won't the obstinate old fool ever listen?'

Stapf and Franz Hartmann exchanged confused glances

'Perhaps you two might have more luck,' Volkmann said.

'More luck at what? Stapf said, trying to calm the big man down.

'The damned apothecaries have been threatening to do something like this for months,' Volkmann ranted, once more ignoring Stapf.

'Like what, Doctor Volkmann?' Stapf urged. 'Sir, please calm down and tell us what has happened.' A young couple walking down the wide promenade hastily skirted the three men obstructing their passage. Automatically, Volkmann tipped the front of his tricorn.

'The apothecaries,' Volkmann said distractedly. 'No doubt

spurred on with glee by the doctors and the university professors.

'The apothecaries ...? The professors ...? What ...? Doctor Volkmann, please. The apothecaries have done what?' Stapf pleaded.

'They've served notice on Hahnemann. The town of Leipzig has received a complaint from the apothecaries accusing Doctor Hahnemann of encroaching upon their privileges by dispensing his own medicine.'

'Oh, my God,' groaned Franz Hartmann.

'I've just seen him to deliver the apothecary's plaint,' Volkmann added, nodding his head to the front door of Hahnemann's rooms.

'What does that mean exactly?' Stapf enquired.

'It means that our good friend will have to defend himself in court. And, perhaps, you as well,' Volkmann said, looking from one man to the other. The apothecaries have been very clear in their written complaint. Their lawyers have no doubt been closely consulted. The complaint expressly reserves the right to name such young medical men who are likewise dispensing their own medicines.'

48

The three Aldermen took their seats behind the bench perched above the proceedings of the court. Intricately carved timber panels surrounded their raised stage, offering protection from the rowdy floor. Elsewhere, the burnished gleam of polished timber added a sombre tone to the proceedings.

Each of the Aldermen wore their robes with the self-importance assured them by their positions with the city. The capes were flecked with ermine; their soft black caps settled easily on their heads; their badge of office hung proudly around their neck, glistening against the fine black cloth at their chest. Sitting in front and slightly below them was Doctor Volkmann, his own robe of office reminding everyone in the court of the Council's authority and of the Town Clerk's legal knowledge.

Samuel glanced across the polished floor separating him from his prosecutors. The three lawyers sat shoulder to shoulder on their allotted bench, papers neatly laid out on the desk in front of them, their robes more subdued in order to give no cause for offence to the magistrates watching over them.

Behind them a solid phalanx of apothecaries sat crammed onto the first bench, their numbers equalled in the row behind. Many of their faces were familiar to Samuel yet their names were hidden in the years. He could not quickly forget the rabid attacks of Rhinehart or Schlutt, or the diminutive Herr Beck. Samuel smiled at the memory of Otto's depiction of the small chairman. Samuel scanned the second row. His eyes fixed on a large man whose familiar face was at odds with his shock of white hair. Recognition came slowly, for surely it was thirty years since he had seen Albert Wagner.

So all my enemies are coming home to roost.

His thoughts were interrupted by a call to order from the Town Clerk, who stood to address the packed court.

'Please rise. The Alderman's Court of the Council of the Town of Leipzig has been convened on this 9th day of February to hear a complaint ...'

The soft murmur from the crowd was immediately cut off. From his solitary position at the front of the court Samuel rose along with the prosecutors and the visitors in the gallery. Out of the corner of his eye he watched the apothecaries stand, each man dressed in his finest, the imported cloths and fancy stitching clashing with the conservative setting. Without needing to turn his head Samuel could picture each of his students, also standing, their lead taken from the calm demeanour of Johann Stapf. Even Franz Hartmann, Samuel had been pleased to see, was considerably calmed from that day in December when Volkmann had delivered the fateful news. 'Was this how it was to be for the rest of our lives? Two opposing factions ranged against each other in a divided court?' Samuel thought.

' ... the complaint has been brought by the Apothecaries of Leipzig, who solemnly claim their rights to be severely and adversely affected by the encroachment of Doctor Christian Friedrich Samuel Hahnemann, by his preparing and dispensing his own medicines in breach of the royal privileges that rule in favour of the pharmacists. Let it be understood that this court acknowledges the rights of the apothecaries to prepare and dispense such compound medicines as being exclusively reserved for them by royal decree.'

Doctor Volkmann looked up from the bill in his hands and cast an eye around the crowded courtroom. Not a single sound broke the silence of the austere chamber.

'Doctor Hahnemann,' Volkmann turned and faced Samuel, 'you have heard the charge made against you. As the court understands it you have decided to provide your own counsel and defend yourself ...' The sudden intake of breath from behind Samuel cut through the silence like a scythe. Volkmann glared at the row of students before continuing. '... against the charges. On behalf of the court I ask how you plead, sir — guilty,' Volkmann paused, 'or not guilty?'

'Unreservedly, not guilty, sir,' Samuel said, his voice carrying clearly throughout the chamber.

A soft murmur rose behind his back, the statement not unexpected by the body of his supporters even though most had had no indication from their mentor of his plans. Only Stapf and the inner circle had been briefed, and each of them was sworn to silence on the strategy to be employed.

Doctor Volkmann turned to the three prosecutors. 'Gentlemen, the Court of Aldermen of the Town of Leipzig recognises your plaint on behalf of the apothecaries of Leipzig and asks that you clearly state your grievance for the court.'

Slowly, the prosecutor sitting on the left of the group rose to his feet, a single sheet of paper in his thin hand, his lean features marked by deep grooves on either side of his face. He nodded at Doctor Volkmann then acknowledged the three Aldermen with a solemn bow of his head. As a courtesy, he looked briefly at Samuel and nodded, pursing his lips. Finally he turned back to address the officials.

'Your Honours, there is really little for me to add to the plaint as lodged. As has been read to the court we are acting on behalf of the industrious and civic-minded apothecaries of our beautiful city who have sought redress against the blatant abuse of their privileges by the defendant, Samuel Hahnemann.'

The prosecutor lifted the sheet of paper in his hand and raised it towards the court. 'Abuse, contrary to the royal decree that has existed in our state for centuries, giving the apothecaries the right to prepare and dispense medicines. A royal decree, I should add, that has gone unchallenged for centuries. We claim that until such a time as the royal decree is withdrawn by his Gracious Majesty, that Doctor Hahnemann and any other physician or student engaged in the study of medicine, and who may, through reasons of their training, be required to diagnose and provide advice to patients on their condition, be compelled to desist from preparing and dispensing medicines under threat of a penalty to be determined by this court.'

The prosecutor stopped; a hint of colour in his face, a sardonic twitch on his lips as he turned to appraise Samuel's reaction.

'Thank you, Doctor Black,' the Alderman seated at the centre of the bench said before turning to his colleagues, each of whom nodded their agreement to proceed. The Alderman turned to face Samuel. 'Doctor Hahnemann, it is my responsibility to preside as president of this Court. However it is our intention,' and with a nod he included both sides, 'to keep these proceedings as informal as possible. We will defer to Doctor Volkmann on any specific point of law that may take us outside the limits of the Council's power, otherwise I intend to offer both the defence and the prosecution the chance to refute the other's statement. I must say also that we have looked closely at the royal mandate and the wording of the memorial appears to my colleagues and I, as being clear and unequivocal. The words specifically state that this is not just a right, vaguely and broadly offered, but the only right, which is exclusively reserved for them.'

The president once more allowed his eyes to range over the crowd in the court. Finally he returned his attention to Samuel, his words laced with conceit. 'Given the specificity of the instructions, I am unsure, sir, what you can say in your defence.'

Despite the murmur that rose behind him, Samuel doggedly kept his eyes locked on the magistrate's, unwilling to allow the blatant attempt to undermine his position to unnerve him. Slowly he gathered himself, calming his beating heart.

'Sir, I take great issue with your opening remark.' Samuel stole a glance at Volkmann, whose expression remained severe.

Samuel continued. 'That it should be inferred that I have little chance of succeeding in my defence suggests at best a preconception of my craft or, at worst, a partiality on the part of the bench towards whatever argument I put forth.'

'How dare you, Doctor Hahnemann,' the president exploded. 'How dare you give directions or make inferences that my colleagues and I will not be impartial. You will need to show far greater care than that, or I promise you I will deal with any transgression with impunity.'

'Sir, if I may.' The gentle interruption came from Doctor Volkmann, who stood and bent forward to whisper to the alderman. After a few moments Volkmann returned to his seat leaving the president with a rising blush of colour on his face.

The alderman tapped the papers in front of him, squaring them against the desk. He cleared his throat. 'Doctor Hahnemann, I, er, please, if you would continue with your defence. We are all busy people. Let us proceed forthwith and without any more digressions. You have my assurance, sir, that this bench will be impartial, and ... we look forward to your deposition.'

Samuel resisted the temptation to look at Volkmann, his eyes locked on the president's.

'Thank you', he acknowledged the president with a bow, 'I am pleased to have such a reassurance as my defence is complex and one that I felt obliged to conduct myself, given the prejudices that my discourse usually touches.'

'Prejudices, Doctor Hahnemann?' The president blustered, before checking himself at a shake of Volkmann's head. 'Surely the courtroom is the place where prejudices can be openly discussed.'

'Quite,' Samuel coughed. 'Your Honours let me be blunt. The method of healing which I use for my patients is quite different from that of other doctors and, consequently, cannot, like theirs, be linked with the work of the apothecaries or, for that matter, to be dependent upon them.'

The president fired a sly glance in Volkmann's direction.

'Doctor Hahnemann, your reputation precedes you. Although I don't profess to understand the intricacies of what you call homeopathy, a person would need to be blind to not be aware of the debate raging in our press and our journals. Like many, I followed the discourse between yourself and the respected Professor Dzondi.' The president hesitated as Volkmann's head turned, the warning in his eye clear. 'Anyway,' the alderman blustered, 'my point is: how can the method of treatment, whether it be hot coals or cold water, have anything to do with it? Simply because you don't agree with another doctor's philosophy surely can't change the need for medicines to assist with the cure.'

'Unfortunately, sir, that is exactly the point of my defence,' Samuel interjected coolly. 'I do not even use the medicines as dispensed by the apothecaries and to which they have the royal monopoly. Furthermore, I argue that the apothecary's privilege is limited to the dispensing of compound medicines, which the allopathic doctor's prescribe meticulously by weight and by price for the apothecary to mix and dispense.' Samuel smiled broadly at his three judges. 'Their argument is even more absurd when you consider the infinitesimally small doses that I prescribe, which would not earn the pharmacist sufficient return to justify the dispensing.'

Bewildered, the president turned to his colleagues, the three men exchanging looks that betrayed their confusion.

'I should add, your worships,' Samuel continued, a smile briefly touching his lips. The three men turned and faced Samuel. 'I too use remedies from nature, but they are only simple drugs not complex compounds such as those covered by the royal decrees. I therefore most emphatically deny encroachment. Besides, I require my remedies only for my own patients, not for sale to other people.'

The president stared at Samuel, the colour in his cheeks rising with his confusion. He looked across at the prosecution table where the three lawyers sat, their eyes locked on the floor in front of them. He looked at the back of the Town Clerk's head. With a deep breath he again turned to Samuel.

'Doctor Hahnemann, I had hoped that this would be a relatively quick proceeding, but clearly you are determined to tease the court with clever words and semantic arguments.'

Doctor Volkmann turned in his seat and glared at the president, who kept his eyes fixed on Samuel, ignoring the warning signals from the Town Clerk.

'We do not intend to sit here,' the president continued, 'and listen to an argument that tries to justify your position on when a drug is not a drug. I intend to adjourn this hearing for five days. In that time, sir, I will expect to receive a written deposition clarifying your defence. I only hope that it contains more than a dissertation on the semantics of what defines a drug.'

49

'Samuel, you must listen to Doctor Volkmann, what he is saying makes complete sense,' Otto Schaefer said, reaching across and pulling at Samuel's sleeve.

Samuel Hahnemann settled back in the comfortable armchair in his study. 'Otto, all I was going to do was offer both of you a light pilsener.'

Otto shrugged in despair at the Town Clerk and released his hold of the sleeve. 'Samuel, why are you so determined to do this without any support or assistance from your friends? It makes no sense.'

'Otto, you were not in the court when the president …' Samuel began.

'And you know perfectly well why, Samuel,' Otto protested. 'I had already left Berlin when I heard. I could not have been here any sooner.'

'Please, my comments were not a criticism,' Samuel said in alarm, laying his hand on Schaefer's arm. 'My comment was to highlight the point that even had I been represented by a battery of lawyers it would have made no difference in that hearing.'

'Doctor, I did try and warn you,' Volkmann said. The aldermen are barely trained as city councillors never mind also being trained in the law. I am there to supposedly give legal advice and opinion but, as you witnessed, they flaunt the rules.'

'I have been meaning to ask, Doctor Volkmann, what did you say to the president at the beginning of the proceedings when he attacked me?'

'I simply reminded him of your rights of appeal, and that we did not need to give you the reason of prejudice on top of any other cause you might find.' Volkmann smiled grimly and turned to Otto. 'I regret that I need to attend a meeting of the aldermen, and cannot remain to help you counsel your friend.' Volkmann fixed his eyes on Samuel. 'If you are going to persist without representation, Doctor Hahnemann, at least allow Herr Schaefer to hear your dissertation and to give you some advice on the tone and manner of your delivery. Please remember, these are not trained lawyers, they are mere mortals whose sense of justice can be swayed by their prejudices, or by, how should I say it, inducements of their city calling.'

50

'If I may be allowed, Your Honour, I would like to begin by quoting from the Latin,' Samuel asked, a tone of respect in his voice. From the raised bench the president nodded his head, one eye watching his Town Clerk.

'*Non debut cui plus licet, quod minus est non licure,*' Samuel began confidently.

'And for those in the court who are not conversant with that language, sir?' the president asked facetiously, his eyebrows raised.

'That which is less, may well be allowed to him to whom more is allowed.'

'I'm sorry ...' the alderman sitting on the right hand side of the bench began. His interruption was waved away by the president.

'Doctor, perhaps we can keep this deposition as simple as possible,' the president responded tersely, his eyebrows raised 'so that everyone in the courtroom can follow your argument.'

Samuel bowed, cursing himself, recalling Otto's caution not to allow his ego to intervene in the proceedings.

'Your Honour,' he mumbled. 'Perhaps then I could start by repeating my assertion that my method of treatment has nothing in common with ordinary medical science. In fact, it is exactly the opposite and, therefore, the existing measurement of medical prescribing can in no way apply.'

'Yes, yes,' replied the chief magistrate. 'I have a clearer picture since we last met. You can be assured we now understand the principles.'

Samuel bowed. 'Thank you, Your Honour. Then I shall continue to elaborate my point regarding the differences between the medicines of the old method and the medicines or remedies we use in homeopathy.' Without waiting for approval, Samuel stepped out from behind the table to address the magistracy and the court at large.

Otto sat at the back, diplomatically midway between the two camps. The front two rows behind the prosecutors were again jammed with the city's apothecaries. To Samuel's right sat a heavy phalanx of his students and a smattering of practicing homeopaths, including Johann Stapf. At the back of the court Samuel recognised a handful of his patients.

'The old method of treatment,' Samuel continued, 'requires what I referred to as compound medicines, each consisting of several ingredients of considerable weight. The compounding of these prescriptions requires skilful, often laborious preparation and takes considerable time. The physician who is busy with his patients does not always have the skill or the time to do this preparation himself. In fact, it could be regarded as dereliction of duty if the physician did this when his time should be devoted to his patients. Therefore the physician calls on an able and well-trained scientific helper — the apothecary — who will prepare these time-wasting and laborious medicinal mixtures, which physicians can prescribe several times a day.'

'Thank you, Doctor Hahnemann, for such a painstaking account of the question of compound medicines,' the president said before turning to the prosecution. 'Do you have any question or comment at this point, Doctor Black?'

The tall, ascetic prosecutor unwound himself and faced the bench. 'Thank you for your consideration, Your Honour. At this stage we have no questions.' The prosecutor resumed his seat, offering a slight bow to Samuel.

'Thank you. Doctor Hahnemann, you may continue.'

Samuel nodded in the direction of the bench. 'Since the very earliest of times, the medical law has always defined dispensing as it applies to the preparation of compound medicines. In the Latin, *ex diversis pensis componere* — *dispensare* literally means to prepare compound medicines in a skilful manner. And nothing else can be implied by it.'

'Your Honour,' the tall prosecutor once again unwound himself from his chair, 'I object to the absolute way in which Doctor Hahnemann uses the Latin and presumes a truth without any evidence to support his statement. I expect at the very least that he would be required to bring before the court an expert who could attest accordingly to the specificity of his translation.'

The president regarded the head prosecutor for a moment. 'Doctor Volkmann, a moment if you please.'

Samuel remained standing while the three aldermen crowded together to consult the Town Clerk. Ten feet away the head prosecutor carefully avoided Samuel's eyes.

The president nodded to Doctor Volkmann and briefly consulted with his two colleagues before returning his attention to the two protagonists. 'On advice, we accept the prosecutor's assertion that verification of the translation will be required if it should later become a point of contention. However, for the moment, we are prepared to allow the comment to stand, as it is part of the submission that we requested of Doctor Hahnemann.'

The head prosecutor inclined his head and returned slowly to his seat.

'Doctor Hahnemann, please continue?' the president prompted gruffly.

'Perhaps I can help clarify the point,' Samuel said gathering his thoughts. 'For as long as I can remember, all the universities, all the medical colleges, as well as all the clinical hospitals, have taught the treatment of disease by requesting their students to make out a prescription. That is, giving the apothecary a list of the medicines he is to combine into one preparation. This is the precedent that has been in place for centuries. Every young physician who presents himself for examination must have studied and acquired the art of writing a prescription containing several medicines for the patient. The right of skilfully preparing these medicines for the training of young students, as it was for the practicing physicians, was exclusively reserved for the apothecaries by royal decree.'

'Thank you, doctor, I think we are clear in our minds about the importance and relevance of compound medicines and the importance of precedent in its evolution.' The president caught the eye of each of his confederates, who nodded. 'Now we would be grateful if you could enlighten us as to why you should be allowed to stand outside this royal decree you acknowledge exists? Because, I suspect, that is where we are going, isn't it?'

Samuel nodded innocently. 'Yes, Your Honour,' he replied. 'Simply put, the new science of treatment that we have called homeopathy has no prescriptions to hand over to the apothecaries.'

'Your Honour, I must object again,' the tall prosecutor held up his hand, this time disdainful of the need to stand. 'Everything we have heard this day is the unsubstantiated commentary of a man who has a vested interest in the tale he is telling. Now we are to believe that this so-called method of treating illness can be effected without the use of medicines. I really must object that without some form of corroboration this is irrelevant.' The prosecutor started to rise. 'And please understand, Your Honour, I am not suggesting that it would not be ... corroborated.' The man was on his feet, turning away from the bench so that he could share his comments with the apothecaries behind him. 'We are taking the opinion of a man who is well-known for his negative attitude towards precedence.' As one, the apothecaries nodded their heads 'With such a low opinion of precedent it is hardly surprising that Doctor Hahnemann would take any other course.' A murmur of assent rose from the gathered apothecaries, earning them a baleful glance from Volkmann and silence from the bench.

Samuel bit back his response, mindful of Otto's caution. He turned his attention to the president whose arms were folded across his chest.

'I must agree, Doctor Hahnemann,' the president finally pronounced. 'I too find it incredible that you would suggest there is a system of medicine that uses no medicine.'

'I have not said there is no medicine, Your Honour,' Samuel interjected angrily. 'If my learned friend had not interrupted he would have heard me explaining that homeopathy does not use compound medicines but only a single, simple remedy for each single case of disease.'

'Doctor, I am becoming heartily tired of hearing about compound medicines,' the president spat back. 'I still don't see how the distinction can change the right of the apothecaries to dispense?'

'Because the word dispensing does not apply.' Samuel gritted his teeth. *Was the alderman being deliberately obtuse, or could he truly not see the point?* He forced himself to remain calm. 'As I have already explained, the word dispensing can only apply to the mixing of compounds; there is no mixing in homeopathy. Thereby the laws which reserve the right for the apothecaries cannot in any form apply to the homeopathic science of treatment.'

This time the tall prosecutor climbed to his feet. 'Your Honour, I really do believe this matter has gone beyond the capacity of the court to make a ruling, even with corroboration. This distinction is becoming tedious. Even the linguists find it hard to agree on many interpretations of our own language, never mind Latin, yet we keep on being dragged back to this same contention that the interpretation only applies to compound medicines, that only compound medicines fit the description of dispensing. From my Latin studies, dispensing is dispensing, no matter how you try to fancy it up.' Slowly the tall prosecutor lowered himself back into his chair. 'Surely, Your Honour, we have heard enough of this. Unless the defendant has something different to add I would urge you to allow all the good people in this court to get about more important business.'

Volkmann rose from his chair and leant across to talk to

the president. With growing alarm, Samuel watched the alderman cross his arms across his chest and shake his head at the Town Clerk. With a resigned look, Volkmann sat down.

'Doctor Hahnemann,' the chief magistrate leant forward, 'I am inclined to agree with the prosecution.' The magistrate cast a baleful glance at the back of the Town Clerk's head. 'So far your case rests very clearly on the Latin distinction, a point that I am still to be convinced about, but which, equally, I am not prepared to have revisited over and over in this court. Unless you have a further point I do believe this court should be adjourned to allow my colleagues and I the opportunity to review the charge.'

Behind Samuel the students let out a sigh of disbelief at the chief magistrate's dismissive tone.

'This is absurd!' Samuel cried out approaching the bench.

'Be careful, sir, or I will hold you in contempt,' the president replied quietly, a sly smile on his lips.

Undeterred, Samuel continued. 'Whether you believe my interpretation of what constitutes a compound or not, whether you are prepared to allow me the chance to put forward experts to support my interpretation or not, there is one thing I can tell you, unequivocally, and which has nothing to do with Latin or German.' Samuel's voice was steadily climbing. 'There is not one mention, not one single syllable in all the royal decrees which forbids a doctor from giving a single remedy to their patient.' Samuel ran a hand across his bald head. 'But even that is not my final word and I demand the right to finish my deposition, whether the learned prosecutor has something better to do or not.'

The tall man began to rise, hesitating at the raised hand of the president.

'You were given this opportunity to make your case, Doctor Hahnemann,' the magistrate said, his voice grim, ' and you shall have the courtesy of the court to finish it.'

Samuel's heart thumped in his chest. He looked at the back of the court where Otto Schaefer held his head in his hands.

Closer to the front he could see Johann Stapf, incredulous at the disdainful, prejudicial tone emanating from the bench.

Samuel straightened his back, rising to his full height. Finally he said, 'I would make two final points, no, three.'

'Well, get on with it then.' The call came from one of the apothecaries, but Samuel was hard pressed to put a face to it.

'Gentlemen, please,' the magistrate held up his hand, a brief smile playing at the corner of his mouth.

Slowly, Samuel took a deep breath. 'For years now, I have taught my students to use only one simple substance to treat their patients. I have successfully applied this principle to some of the most dangerous diseases known to man, and have effected a cure. Not only have I followed the principle of one substance, I have argued that only the smallest, infinitesimally small, dosage of each single remedy should be given. By this practice I have eliminated any danger to the patient from the medicine itself whilst, through the mysteries of chemistry, I have succeeded in increasing the medicine's potency.' Again Samuel paused to collect his thoughts. 'Sir, my record speaks for itself, yet the apothecaries ridicule these medicines because of their supposed lack of substance but, I suspect, the reason is much closer to their pecuniary god than to our Father in Heaven, who must look down sadly on the poor victims of our doctors and apothecaries and wince as He watches their bellies being stuffed full of unnecessary potions.'

'Why don't you take your witchcraft to another planet, Hahnemann.' The shout again came from amongst the group of apothecaries.

'Gentlemen.' Volkmann rose angrily to his feet. 'I will have the next man who interrupts ejected from this court. Am I understood, Herr Rhinehart?' The Town Clerk resumed his seat, unaware of the smile that had flashed across the president's face.

Samuel's heart thudded harder, that single smile worse than any sentence.

'Thank you, Doctor Volkmann,' the president added ponderously. 'Any further interruptions will not be tolerated. I apologise, Doctor Hahnemann, but perhaps you would be good enough to finish your point.'

Samuel swallowed, taking the time to compose himself. 'My point is that in their correct form most of the remedies used in homeopathy cannot be detected unless they are dispensed under the physician's own watchful eye. And as we have witnessed in this courtroom, the apothecaries do not endear themselves to the homeopath. In turn, homeopaths have little reason to trust that the apothecaries will dispense with the level of accuracy so critical to our cure.' Samuel reached across to the water jug on his table and filled a tumbler with water.

'That is the first point I wish to make,' Samuel continued. 'The second, and I say this for the benefit of all the apothecaries gathered here, the homeopath does not represent a threat to you as a vendor of medicines as we don't charge for the infinitely small dose of the single remedy we dispense. Instead we give it to the patient freely, and take reimbursement for our labours in researching the nature of our patient's condition or disease.'

A roar erupted from the apothecaries.

Samuel took a sip of water, determined to finish. 'My final argument has nothing to do with the past, but is a plea to the future.' Samuel took a second sip and fixed his eyes on the three aldermen. 'Homeopathy has already proven itself to be of enormous benefit to the people of Leipzig and to all of Saxony. It has cured typhus, and has cured many of the people in this room who had despaired at their lack of progress under the so-called healing power of the doctors and apothecaries.' Without interruptions Samuel's confidence began to return. 'If you take away the right of homeopaths to dispense their own remedies, then you will effectively sound a death knell for this new science of healing. I ask that this court insist that the apothecaries of Leipzig be compelled to remain within the limits of their own privileges and be cautioned that their authority does not extend to this new art of healing.'

Exhausted, Samuel bowed his head towards the bench and returned to his seat, carefully placing the water tumbler on the table. An angry murmur came from the apothecaries.

The president nodded to Samuel before turning to consult each of his colleagues. The noise from the crowd grew louder. The president turned to face the court, but before he could speak Samuel rose abruptly from his chair. 'Your Honour, with the court's indulgence?'

The chief magistrate blinked at the unexpected intrusion. 'Yes, Doctor Hahnemann, is there something you would like to add?'

'Yes, Your Honour,' Samuel rejoined, wringing his hands together. 'I apologise, but in the emotion of my conclusion there is something in the complaint that I have not responded to.'

'It seems to me that you have responded in the extreme. Your reply could well be described as tedious.'

Samuel's face flushed bright red. 'There is the issue, Your Honour, of my students.'

'Your students? I fail to see what your students have to do with this?'

Volkmann quickly rose to his feet and leaned across to whisper to the president, who in turn nodded his head.

'Ah, I think I understand your concern, Doctor Hahnemann,' the president said, 'the legal reference reserving the rights of the apothecaries to name other doctors and students also dispensing medicines. Well, sir, what do you wish to say?'

'Only this. As far as my pupils are concerned, I am not in any way connected with them, and since they are all of a strong calibre I do not need to represent them.' Behind him Samuel could hear the cries of surprise from his students. Rigidly he continued to face the bench. 'I consider no man my disciple beholden to me or requiring supervision from me. And I believe that only men of strong moral character would choose to practice this new science and that they will know that the remedies they administer to their patients contain so small a dose of the medicinal substance that they can do no harm to the patient. Such a minute dosage negates the necessity of exercising official supervision and care on the part of the teacher or authorities.'

'I'm not sure I quite understand the point you are making,

Doctor Hahnemann, other than to reinforce those you have already made.'

'What I am saying is very simple. If the student is wel-trained in the principles of diagnosis, the question of dispensing is an irrelevancy. The medicines we use are of no danger to anyone except the apothecary's pocket. And I will not allow the reputation of homeopathy to be sullied by bad practice or by charlatans wishing to capitalise on the fast-spreading good name of the science. Nor should homeopathy be branded a fake because of the avarice and greed of the apothecaries, who are unable to see the importance of simple remedies.'

Samuel heard the rumblings from the opposite side of the room but held his resolve. 'Ultimately, every student must be his own judge and jury as to his dedication to the science. If that is held true, homeopathy will flourish for the benefit of mankind. If other motivations and controls appear under the cloak of homeopathy, then it cannot survive and will languish through its failure to heal.'

Out of the corner of his eye Samuel saw a burly figure seated behind the prosecutor climb to his feet.

'You arrogant bastard, Hahnemann.' Albert Wagner raised his fist and waved it at Samuel. 'This time you've gone too far. If this court hasn't the balls to put an end to you, I'll have you for defamation. God knows I've got the witnesses.'

As pandemonium erupted in the court, Samuel rocked on his heels, stunned at the hatred and bitterness in Wagner's words.

51

'Doctor Volkmann, perhaps you can explain the implications of the court's ruling,' Johann Stapf asked. The doctor sat in a hard-backed chair in front of the Town Clerk's desk. Beside him, Franz Hartmann crossed one leg over the other trying to find a comfortable position.

'Have you spoken to Doctor Hahnemann?' Volkmann replied, his hands resting on the leather inlay.

'Not since the judgement was handed down.'

'Delivered to his home, more precisely,' observed Hartmann.

'Careful, Doctor Hartmann,' Volkmann chided the young man, 'as the one responsible for that dubious honour I have a certain sensitivity to such retorts.'

Hartmann blushed but continued doggedly, 'The last word we had with the good doctor was two weeks ago, before the judgement. I have never seen him at such a low ebb.'

'Does he still see his patients?' Volkmann asked.

This time it was Stapf who answered. 'Some. He has refused to take new patients.'

'He is just going through the motions,' Franz Hartmann added. 'He spends no time on small talk, asking his questions in a perfunctory manner, quickly moving on to his next patient. He has also cancelled his lectures.'

'Postponed, Franz, not cancelled,' Stapf interjected. 'We must be careful not to give the wrong impression.' Stapf turned to the Town Clerk. 'As he will not talk to us, we have no way of forming our plans. That is why we have come to you. If we can understand what is to happen we can consider our next steps.'

'Unfortunately the ruling is absolutely clear. He should cease the distributing and dispensing of any and every medicine, to anybody, or face a penalty of 20 thaler. It closes by warning Doctor Hahnemann to give no cause for more severe regulations.'

'More severe?' Hartmann gasped. 'Twenty thaler is penalty enough. The good aldermen of the town must be in serious need of funds for the council's works.'

Volkmann glared at the young man before addressing his next remarks to Stapf. 'The decree does not come into effect until the state confirms it. So until that time, Doctor Hahnemann and the rest of you are free to continue dispensing your remedies and curing people.'

Stapf nodded his understanding. 'When do you expect the decree to be recognised by the state?'

Volkmann smiled grimly. 'In just over seven months, the 30th of November to be precise.'

'And then?' Stapf asked.

'Then? Expect to be fined 20 thaler each time you dispense a remedy in Leipzig.'

'And outside Leipzig?'

'The Town Council and the aldermen's court has limited power, Doctor Stapf,' the Town Clerk replied. 'But ...'

'But ...?' Hartmann inquired.

'But you would have to be very naïve if you believed that this little court case hasn't sparked interest in other parts.'

'Do we have any right of appeal on behalf of Doctor Hahnemann?' Stapf said, 'and of course for ourselves.'

'You could write to the king. Naturally he has the power to overrule the council, though he very rarely does,' Volkmann observed with a grim smile. 'Could I make a suggestion,

Doctor Stapf?'

'Of course.' Stapf looked at Hartmann and then returned his attention to Volkmann. 'We would be grateful for any guidance.'

'During the second day of the court case, I noticed Otto Schaefer. I understand he is a close confidante of Doctor Hahnemann, and yet he is a practicing apothecary isn't he?' Stapf nodded. 'Surely the way to move forward is to nurture your relationships with some of the younger apothecaries, in much the same way as Doctor Hahnemann has nurtured the younger students.'

Hartmann leant forward, his eyebrows reaching his hairline.

'Oh, don't be so surprised, young Hartmann, there are still some people in the world who don't walk around with their eyes closed,' Volkmann said before returning his attention to Johann Stapf. 'Clearly Doctor Hahnemann and Schaefer have formed a close bond that has withstood the pressures of conflicting interests.'

'Yes, and Otto has also given wise counsel on the way to try and satisfy the interests of the apothecaries and the homeopaths. Unfortunately the mistrust runs so deep it is difficult to see who would take a lead in such a massive undertaking. The two things are so philosophically at odds,' Stapf said wearily and then spread his hands. 'I suspect that no matter how willing the homeopaths may be we will not find many apothecaries with the same tolerance as Otto Schaefer, or with the same *laissez-faire* approach to money.' Stapf finished with a sad smile.

The burly Town Clerk rose to his feet and held out his hand to Johann Stapf. 'Well, unless you can find a way to work with the apothecaries I have to warn you that by Christmas you will have little reason to celebrate.'

52

The tall gentlemen standing on the doorstep removed his tricorn and bowed deeply to Johanna Hahnemann. 'Madam, my name is Joseph Edler von Sax, physician to His Royal Highness Prince Karl of Schwarzenberg.'

Johanna took a small step back. The hawk-like features of the visitor stared back at her from an equal level, even though he stood a good step below her.

'I have come to pay my respects to your husband on behalf of his Royal Highness, who wishes the good doctor to visit with him as a possible patient.'

'His Royal Highness? I'm sorry, my husband has recently been ... er ... has indicated that he no longer intends to take new patients.'

'Madam, I fear this is a matter of the utmost urgency, perhaps even of life and death. May I politely insist that I be taken to your husband?'

Johanna shook her head, her confusion earning a stern scowl from the man standing in the street. Flustered, Johanna stepped aside. 'Please, Doctor ...?'

'von Sax.'

'Come in Doctor von Sax, I will show you to my husband's waiting room. But please understand I cannot promise that he will agree to see you. The town's council has recently prosecuted him. The judgement was only handed down a month ago and he is still ... he is still in a state of some shock.'

'von Sax?' The tall visitor looked up from the copy of *Hufeland's Journal* he was reading. Samuel stood in the doorway to his waiting room. 'I understand you wish to see me?'

'Yes, thank you. It is a privilege.' von Sax rose from his chair and held out his hand.

'Can we get to business, doctor,' Samuel said ignoring the outstretched hand. 'I am well aware of your opinion of me and of your relationship with von Stifft, the so-called trusted adviser to Emperor Franz. It is common knowledge that the two of you were up to your eyeballs in persuading his majesty to ban the practice of homeopathy in Austria.'

'I must protest.' Unconsciously von Sax ran a finger around the inside of his heavily starched collar, 'von Stifft asked me for an opinion and I gave it, nothing more. I think you do me a disservice, sir. I have come here to ask you if you would be prepared to attend His Royal Highness, who has already written to you asking that you treat him.'

'And I replied at the time that I could not possibly desert my existing patients and travel to Austria to do so.' Samuel turned from his visitor. 'Anyway,' he said resignedly, 'it is now a moot point. My position has changed since we last corresponded. I am not taking new patients, and even if I were I would still not be prepared to desert those who I am treating to visit Austria and treat the prince.'

'I think you miss the point of your own criticism, Doctor Hahnemann,' von Sax said primly. 'Since the Emperor banned homeopathy you would not be welcome in our country to treat the prince. That is why Prince Karl has insisted on being brought here to Leipzig to be treated by you.'

'Doctor Hahnemann,' von Sax waved a hand, 'allow me to introduce Doctor Marenzeller, the regimental doctor.' Samuel shook Marenzeller's hand, appraising the fresh-faced doctor who in his middle years still maintained a shock of dark brown hair and bushy muttonchops.

'I am honoured, Doctor Hahnemann. I have praised your work to no avail in my homeland. Perhaps one day we will again see the light,' Marenzeller said, a twinkle in his eye.

'You are very kind, sir. I must admit it was a sad day for me when my philosophies were so savagely treated by your King.'

'Don't be so harsh on the Emperor, Doctor Hahnemann,' the twinkle in Marenzeller's eye shone brightly, 'he is not a medical man and must rely on the recommendations of others.'

'You should keep a civil tongue in your head, Marenzeller,' snapped von Sax. 'Don't get above your station, sir. I am still the Royal Physician in this household, whether it be at this wretched estate or in the comfort of our own palace.'

Samuel looked around the drawing room, acknowledging the opulence of the fittings without being able to name the craftsmen or the painters of the portraits hanging on the heavily panelled walls. 'It seems to me, von Sax,' he said, 'that half of Leipzig could find comfort here in Milkisle. I live only a few miles from such grandeur but have never even been invited onto the grounds of this magnificent estate.'

'It will serve our purposes no doubt,' observed von Sax brusquely. The tall doctor clapped his hands. 'We are wasting time, Marenzeller, why don't you appraise Hahnemann of the prince's current condition.'

'I would prefer to ask the prince the state of his own condition,' Samuel said quietly. 'Perhaps if I could be shown to his chamber?'

Marenzeller inclined his head to von Sax.

'Very well,' von Sax said, dismissing the two men with another wave of his hand. 'Take Doctor Hahnemann to the prince. Perhaps he will allow you to give him some of the details as you go.' With that said the tall doctor turned on his heel and left.

'I gather von Sax is not pleased to have me here.' Samuel

said with a grim smile.

'Fortunately it is the prince's wishes that matter, and he is a keen advocate for your methods.'

'I had no idea ...'

'In many ways the prince is an extremely astute man. In others ...? Well ...'

'Please, Doctor Marenzeller, I cannot work when I am surrounded by riddles.'

Marenzeller smiled. 'Those who spoke highly of you also warned that you could be ... prickly. Yes, that is the word. There is no riddle,' Marenzeller said, his manner once again serious. 'The prince is well-known as a heavy drinker. Fortunately his exploits on the battlefields have gained him more press than his carousing in the wine cellars and inns of Europe.'

'From my experience heavy drinking would not be the cause of the stroke, although it is without doubt a contributing factor.' Samuel shook his head. 'How long has the prince suffered?'

'He had the stroke on the 13th of January, three years ago. The stroke left him paralysed down the right side. There have been subsequent attacks of paralysis followed by lengthy periods of lethargy. He is a strong man and has regained some of the use of his body through constant exercise but the effects are still severe. The worst part of it is the insomnia he has suffered since the first stroke.'

'He gets no sleep?'

'Very little,' Marenzeller replied. 'I had a concern that he wouldn't even have the strength to climb out of his sick bed to make the journey here.'

'But obviously he has done so, and survived.'

'Come, I will take you to meet the prince. You will find him an ardent admirer.'

Samuel felt for the prince's pulse. It was strong but slightly fast. He leant back and inspected his new patient. Prince Karl was propped up in bed, several pillows supporting his back. Samuel could see the slightly withered state of the man's right arm, which was at odds with the power still evident in the man's upper torso. 'What is your diet, your majesty?' Samuel asked.

Prince Karl smiled, the effect lop-sided due to the paralysis on his right side. A thin line of saliva marked his chin, taking Samuel's attention from the bushy muttonchops that rivalled Marenzeller's for splendour.

'My diet,' the prince wiped the spittle from the side of his mouth with a cloth. 'If yew mean, am I sthill drinking, the ansher is no.' The prince smiled at his own humour. 'Thees people won't 'low me s'much's a sniff.' Prince Karl nodded at Marenzeller.

'No, I was referring more to your food intake than to the amount of alcohol you may be consuming. Although I'm pleased to hear that your physicians have restricted your imbibing.'

'You may be, doctor, I'm not so shuur.'

'Then you may be even less impressed when I describe the diet I propose to place you on.' Samuel smiled at the prince. 'But I have no doubt that with homeopathy we can give you much more pleasure in your life than you are currently enjoying.'

53

Otto Schaefer warmly embraced Johann Stapf and then shook hands with Franz Hartmann. 'It is very good to see you both. Let's order breakfast then you can tell me how it goes with Samuel.' Schaefer waved the two men in the direction of a table in the corner of the inn's dining room.

Johann Stapf caught the eye of the innkeeper's daughter, who had blossomed into an attractive, buxom young woman who enjoyed flirting with the dark brooding doctor from Naumberg.

'The usual?' Stapf asked. He winked at the woman as Otto nodded contentedly, patting his stomach with obvious relish. Stapf turned to Hartmann, 'Franz, I'd get your order in quickly before the pantry is cleaned out.'

Otto rubbed his hands together in fond anticipation. 'I really don't understand how the pair of you survive. Neither of you eats enough to satisfy a mouse, never mind busy doctors.'

'Almost a doctor, Herr Schaefer,' Hartmann said. 'Unfortunately Dean Rosenmüller passed away before I could sit my *viva voce*.'

'Surely you reapplied?' Otto asked.

'Not quite that simple,' Stapf interrupted. 'Our young friend was roundly abused by a doctor for prescribing homeopathic medicines to one of this fellow's patients.'

'So? There is no law against that. At least not until November,' Otto said, his attention distracted by the kitchen door bursting open.

Stapf followed his friend's gaze, smiling at the sight of the heaped platter of food on the waitress's shoulder. He nudged his young friend in the arm. 'Stand by, Franz, you are in for a culinary lesson you will never forget.'

'I fear that's a trifle exaggerated, Stapf,' Otto said indignantly, returning his attention to his two companions. 'And I still don't see how one doctor's rivalry could be considered damning to Hartmann's cause?'

'The doctor took the matter to Clarus,' Hartmann replied. 'As I was still under the jurisdiction of the university, he prosecuted me. Barred me from taking the exam.'

'The bastard,' Otto sneered. 'So go elsewhere and sit the *viva voce*.'

'I applied to Berlin. Unfortunately they had closed their intake.'

'Come to Dresden,' Otto cried. 'I will personally introduce you to the Dean, who is now one of my most delighted customers. And prompt with his bill. No favours, mind, you sit it fair and square.'

'That is most generous of you,' Hartmann replied. 'I have already applied here in Leipzig and am currently awaiting the university's instructions. However I promise you, Herr Schaefer, if they reject me one more time I will take you up on your offer.'

'Good!' Otto rubbed his hands together, his mouth drooling at the array of food in front of him. 'Now that we have that out of the way, perhaps you will be so good as to tell me what has been happening to Samuel. What news is there of Schwarzenberg?'

'I'm sure you already know about the prince, Otto,' Stapf responded. 'But to humour you, I can tell you that Samuel has worked a miracle. Inside three months he now has the man out of his bed for extended periods every day. The paralysis on his right side has eased dramatically, although it is unlikely to ever be gone completely.' Stapf broke open a roll and reached for the butter. 'We all realise it would be foolhardy to get over confident just yet, but the signs are very encouraging. Wouldn't you agree, Franz?'

'Most assuredly,' Hartmann said. 'I visited the prince with Doctor Hahnemann and my close friend, Christian Hornburg, only last week.' Hartmann offered a broad smile in response to the apothecary's raised eyebrow. 'It would appear that the prince's own physicians have tired a little of Doctor Hahnemann's tirades and appreciate our tempering influence on the good doctor.' His voice resumed a serious tone. 'There is no doubt that the prince has improved. His slurred speech will never be perfect but he has made significant gains in that regar''. He also continues to build strength in his arms and legs — very encouraging to say the least.'

'And what of Samuel?' Otto asked between mouthfuls.

'Franz Hartmann shook his head. 'He barely speaks. Since the apothecaries challenged him he seems only intent on biding his time until the state ratifies the decision. Then I fear he will pack his bags and retire to Meissen.'

'Otto shook his head sadly. 'Damn Wagner and his cronies.' Otto reached out and grasped a small, sweet roll. 'What time did you say we are expected, Johann?'

'At eleven. Caroline has promised me that she will make sure he stays home.'

'What does he do with his time if he has reduced his patient load?'

'He walks in the countryside. Some days he sits in his study and reads.'

'The bastards,' said Otto Schaefer, and popped the sweet roll into his mouth.

'Come in, gentlemen. Uncle Otto, you look happy and replete.' Caroline leant forward and kissed the portly apothecary on the cheek, winking at Franz Hartmann over his shoulder.

'You are particular cheery this morning, Caroline,' Hartmann said, returning her smile.

'Well, if you would hurry up and come in off the street I could give you a hint as to why.'

Schaefer accepted Caroline's offer of help to remove his overcoat while the two young doctors exchanged glances.

'And you two gentlemen, can I hang your coats also?' Caroline asked.

Hurriedly they removed their coats and passed them to Caroline, who hung them on pegs beside the rag taggle collection already there.

'Well, are you going to tell us what is going on or will you keep us in suspense for eternity?' Hartmann asked the young woman.

'I think I should allow father that pleasure ...'

Suddenly the study door flew open and Samuel Hahnemann stood in the doorway.

'So you are the cause of all this noise,' the elderly doctor said sternly. 'I should have known.' Suddenly he turned and walked back into his study, leaving the three men to exchange surprised looks.

'Are you going to stand in the passage all day or come in and meet my guest?' Samuel called from inside his study.

Otto Schaefer nodded his thanks to Caroline and walked through the door, followed by Hartmann and Stapf. A dour Samuel Hahnemann and another man greeted them, the newcomer's bushy muttonchops failing to hide the broad smile on his face.

'Doctor Marenzeller!' Franz Hartmann cried out. 'What has ...? Is the prince all right?'

'It is not bad news that I bring, young man. Quite the contrary, the prince is gaining strength daily.'

'Otto, Stapf.' Samuel stepped between his two good friends and grasped each man's arm. 'Allow me to introduce my guest before young Franz has a heart attack.' Samuel smiled at Hartmann. 'Doctor Marenzeller is the regimental doctor attending Prince Karl of Schwarzenberg and, I should add, a good friend of homeopathy. Doctor, this is Johann Stapf, from Naumberg and Otto Schaefer, formerly of Leipzig now domiciled in Dresden.'

Samuel spoke as the three men shook hands. 'The doctor has brought some interesting news and I am delighted to be able to share it with you.' Expectantly the new arrivals waited for Samuel to continue.

'It would appear that young men can't hold their tongues.' Samuel looked accusingly at Franz Hartmann, a hint of a smile tugging at his lips. 'Apparently Doctors Hartmann and Hornburg have been currying favour with the prince behind my back.'

Johann Stapf gave his young friend a quick glance, bewilderment creasing his brow.

'It would appear,' Samuel continued, 'that the prince was particularly interested in knowing more about my time in the aldermen's court, a tale that Hornburg apparently took great delight in recounting. Perhaps, Doctor Marenzeller, you would be good enough to complete the story.'

'With pleasure.' Doctor Marenzeller reached into his pocket and pulled out an envelope. The three newcomers could see the seal of His Majesty, King Friedrich of Saxony, on the back of the folded parchment. 'I have here, gentlemen, a letter signed by King Friedrich and addressed to Prince Karl of Schwarzenberg. You may recall that His Highness was the prince's prisoner after the Battle of Leipzig. He also happens to be the prince's cousin.'

'King Friedrich?' Franz said open-mouthed.

'Yes,' Marenzeller smiled. 'I feel I should digress ... just for a moment,' he added hurriedly seeing the expressions on the faces of his audience. 'For three years I have been beside the sick bed of the prince, ever since his stroke. That such a great man, and such a great leader, should be stricken down in his prime is a tragedy.' Around him the four men shook their heads gravely. 'I was particularly keen for the prince to be treated homeopathically. Unfortunately my colleagues believe in much stronger measures so it was only when their endeavours had been exhausted that I had any chance to put forward my suggestion. The prince had also heard much about Doctor Hahnemann's methods and was very keen for us to secure his services. Some time ago we wrote to Doctor Hahnemann ...'

'I remember you telling me, Samuel,' Otto Schaefer interrupted. 'When was that — a year ago?'

'At least, Otto,' Samuel replied, smiling warmly at his friend.

'So far it would appear that your decision and your Lord's have been vindicated,' Johann Stapf observed.

'Very much so.' The Regimental Surgeon suddenly remembered the folded parchment in his hands. He smiled. 'I promised I would not digress for too long. I mentioned that Prince Karl was also a cousin of the king?' Marenzeller looked around the group, each man nodding his head. 'Well, the prince wrote to the king requesting that he intervene in the matter of the decree by the aldermen's court that threatens to prevent Doctor Hahnemann from treating patients homeopathically. This, gentlemen, is the king's reply.'

The three newcomers stared at each other, stunned by Marenzeller's announcement.

'Well, what does it say?' Otto finally blustered. 'What does it say?'

'Perhaps you would bear with me if I read it,' Marenzeller said unfolding the parchment. He coughed to clear his throat. 'The colonel, Baron Wernhardt ...'

'Wernhardt is a trusted aide of the prince,' interjected Hartmann for the benefit of his two colleagues.

'Thank you, Doctor Hartmann,' Marenzeller smiled, then proceeded to read the letter. 'The colonel, Baron Wernhardt, whom you have sent, has already delivered your message in connection with the matter of Doctor Hahnemann of Leipzig and has received from me an answer to the effect that I shall make enquiries. I have ordered all that is necessary for that to be done and have arranged, at the same time, that no further steps shall be taken against Doctor Hahnemann. In any case, he shall not be hindered in his efforts to cure your dear person with his new method of treatment.' Marenzeller lifted his eyes from the letter and regarded Samuel's colleagues. 'It is signed, Your affectionate friend, Friedrich, King of Saxony.'

54

'It has been a monumental day, Samuel, to say the least.'
'Colossal, Otto, one might even say epic.'

The two men sat in Samuel's study, a glass of pilsener in front of each of them.

'Had you any inkling that this was coming?' Otto Schaefer asked his friend.

Samuel shook his head. 'Absolutely none. The prince never said a word about his intentions. I was aware of the family connection. It intrigued me. Ever since the Battle of Leipzig it has saddened me that so many families were split by the war, that our King should be related to our enemy. Then in a blink of an eye our enemy became our friend and our King became a prisoner in his own land.'

'You are beginning to ramble, my old friend,' Otto warned, smiling warmly.

'Then old must be the telling word. Ever since the court's decision I have felt weary, weary to the bone.' Samuel closed his eyes, massaging his forehead with his fingers. He looked up at his friend, moisture clouding his eyes. Angrily he rubbed them with the heels of his palms.

'Your friends never deserted you,' Otto pointed out gently.

'I know, but I could not bring myself to face them. All my life I have tried to help others, whether through my translations or my obsession to prove the truth of homeopathy. Yet for all my good purpose I found myself hauled before the court, not because what I was trying to achieve could help others but because what I was doing didn't help some. I'm sorry, Otto, because I know, in a way, that also attacks you.'

A deep sigh broke from Otto's lips. 'And there is your problem, Samuel. Right there in those few words.'

Surprised, Samuel waited for his friend to continue.

'How many years have we been friends?' Otto shook his head. 'After all these years you cannot believe that first and foremost I am your friend ... and then I am an apothecary. If the truth be known, I'm not even a very good apothecary these days, more like a freight agent.' He smiled grimly. 'All the people who you have mentored have stayed loyal to you to the very last. Even after you appeared to denounce them in the court they understood that you were placing the principles of homeopathy above everything.' The portly apothecary shook his head, blinking away the tears in his eyes. 'Samuel, when will you understand that your family, your friends and all of your patients love you because of your principles, because of what you believe in and fight for. Yet when those people needed you most, when they needed to be reassured that the fight was not lost ... you deserted them. You closed the door in their faces because you believed they would see you as the failure.'

For a moment Otto watched as his old friend blinked away tears. 'Samuel, the only failure in that court was the system. Prince Karl doesn't see you as a failure, regardless of what may happen. Johann Stapf doesn't see you as a failure; he has seen the proof of your beliefs in the cure of his own patients. Young men like Hartmann and Hornburg don't fight the system in order that they should gain your respect, they fight the system because you have instilled in them similar beliefs to your own, that the people deserve better and that the system is letting them down. Just like the system let you down.' Otto reached over and picked up his glass of pilsener. 'Enough! There has been too much sentimentality. Isn't it about time we took the prince's lead and got back into the fray?'

55

Samuel alighted from the landau, tipping his tricorn to the driver. The day was perfect, the warmth of the late summer sun easing the touch of stiffness in his shoulder. The smell of freshly cut grass drifted across the wide gravel forecourt of the estate. Behind him he heard the crunch of the coach on the crushed stone as it moved away. Three men waited on the broad steps leading up to Milkisle. He was delighted to see Prince Karl with the two doctors, his lopsided grin cheering Samuel's heart.

'Prince Karl, what a pleasure to see you enjoying the sunlight.' Samuel called out, delighted to see the grin widen. He nodded at von Sax, who returned the greeting perfunctorily, then Samuel smiled warmly at Marenzeller, who had one hand held lightly under the prince's elbow.

'Have you had your exercise yet, your lordship?' Samuel asked.

'Not yet,' Prince Karl replied, still smiling broadly. 'I had hoped we could share that pleasure.'

Samuel nodded in approval as Marenzeller guided the prince down the last few steps. He marvelled at the recovery of the man since April.

He is still wasted in his body, Samuel observed, but that will improve if his health holds.

Samuel reached out and gently grasped the prince's elbow, steering him in the direction of the lawn where large ash and elm trees had been planted to provide an avenue of shade. Slowly they crossed the gravel, the soft crunch replaced by the manicured lushness of the grass.

'I remember as if it were only yesterday, the afternoon you rode triumphantly into Leipzig. I was standing in the Burgstrasse. You actually looked me in the eye and saluted.'

Prince Karl shook his head. 'What a shambles of a battle that was. I swore never again to be General and F ...ffield Marshall for a spoiled bunch of kings.'

The two men walked a few paces in silence, enjoying the cool shade of the trees.

'How goes the battle, Doctor Hahnemann?' Prince Karl asked.

'You are the better judge of that than I, my lord,' Samuel replied.

'I wasn't ref ...ferring to my health, good sir,' again the lopsided grin came out, 'more to your battle with the apof ...ffecaries.'

Samuel pursed his lips. 'Oh, that fight. I'm not sure that I am winning too many battles, my lord.'

Prince Karl raised an enquiring eyebrow.

'I have resumed my lectures and my loyal students continue their industry, but there are very few other takers. The university has taken to persecuting any of my students who step out of line. None of them dares miss any of their other lectures, knowing that Clarus will swoop on them like a hawk.'

'Even a hawk has its vulnerability's, doctor.'

'Yes, I understand, and the students are certainly learning how to be more nimble and agile. We also have friends in places where we need them, like the council.'

'And your patients?' the prince prompted.

'Yes, but only to a point. Unless they have influential friends the medical fraternity simply flattens any opposition. We have taken the advice of my good friends Otto Schaefer and Doctor

Volkmann. Both men have urged us to explore whether the hatred of the apothecaries is total or whether there are some members who will agree that the welfare of the patient should be their overriding priority.'

'With any success?'

'Some of the younger apothecaries will open their minds to the argument. It is very hard to change beliefs and practices that have been in place for centuries.'

'Yet we all have to accept change, doctor,' Prince Karl urged. 'F... for accuracy and distance the longbow will outshoot any musket, but it takes years to train an archer, whereas an infantryman can be trained to use a musket in a matter of hours.'

'I understand that change is inevitable, my lord, but, using your analogy, convenience is the friend of the apothecary and the enemy of the homeopath. And winning over the apothecaries is, of course, only part of the battle.'

'Men like von Sax you mean.'

Samuel nodded. 'Doctors, like some generals, rule mostly from fear. They threaten their patients with unknown perils that only they, the doctors, can deal with. They prescribe so-called cures for these perils that the patient must take on trust. What other option do they have when they don't have the training that the doctor has received? That's the way medicine has been delivered for centuries. That I seek to change their view is most clearly a threat, not just to their livelihood but also to their ingrained training. Even men like Clarus, charged with the terrible responsibility of teaching our young doctors, use fear to maintain their hold.'

'Then you must redouble your ef..fforts, Doctor Hahnemann. Having gained you a stay of execution I am determined to see you continue to take the f..ffight to the enemy.'

The two men completed their slow circuit, returning to the steps at the front of the manor house. Marenzeller waited at the top. A manservant stood patiently behind a wheelchair. As the man wheeled Prince Karl back into the house, Marenzeller caught Samuel's arm.

'A moment if you will, before you conduct your examination.'

'Certainly, Doctor Marenzeller,' his smile slipping at the downcast expression on his colleague's face.

'I wanted to alert you to a change in the prince's diet. I considered it prudent to tell you out of earshot of Doctor von Sax.'

'What sort of change? Samuel asked, alarmed.

'Hopefully nothing too serious, but von Sax is permitting the prince to imbibe a little wine each night.'

'Only wine?' Samuel said, relaxing slightly.

Marenzeller nodded. 'At this stage.'

56

'Quickly doctor,' the prince's coachman pleaded as he opened the door. Samuel stepped out of the coach while pulling his cloak around him against the chill in the autumn air. Anxiously the driver handed Samuel his bag, closing the door behind him. 'Doctor Marenzeller said he would wait for you in the drawing room.' The driver waved his hand at the servant waiting for them. 'Schmidt will show you.'

Samuel nodded at the footman who stood silhouetted against the lights at the front of the house. 'Thank you,' he said to the driver. Beside him the footman offered to take his bag. Samuel shook his head and walked briskly across the short expanse of gravel to the steps.

Marenzeller greeted Samuel at the front door, wringing his hands. 'Thank you for coming at this time of night.'

'What is happening? The coachman was very evasive. All he would say was that the prince had had some sort of relapse.'

The regimental doctor nodded anxiously. 'I will be blunt. The prince has slipped steadily into his old ways. You will remember the last time I saw you I advised that the prince was imbibing a little wine with his dinner?'

Samuel inclined his head. 'You said it was only wine, and in small amounts, I had no problem with that. Are you saying that in the space of a month the prince has reverted to his heavy drinking?'

Marenzeller nodded. 'And not just wine. He instructs the servants to bring him his favourite whiskey and starts drinking before lunch.'

'Why hasn't someone instructed the servants to desist, or to even clear the stuff out of the house?'

'Because he has ordered them not to.'

'What do you mean, ordered them? May I remind you that the prince is currently under doctor's orders — my orders.' Samuel turned and began to walk to the broad stairway that led to the prince's quarters.

At the base of the stairs Samuel stopped and looked over his shoulder. Marenzeller hadn't moved.

'What is it, man?' Samuel asked gruffly.

The regimental doctor wrung his hands. 'Doctor Hahnemann, I must warn you that I was the one who took the decision to ask you here tonight. Contrary to von Sax's instructions.'

'What do you mean, contrary to his instructions?' Samuel asked, a baffled look on his face. 'Who is with the prince now?'

'von Sax.'

'Only von Sax?'

'Well,' Marenzeller hesitated, 'von Sax and several physicians from Leipzig who von Sax has invited to give another opinion.'

'He's asked them to do what?' shouted Samuel. 'Has anyone asked the prince if he wants another opinion?'

Samuel scaled the stairs three at a time, Marenzeller keeping pace with him. At the doorway to the prince's bedroom Samuel paused to catch his breath. He grasped the doorknob and flung the door open wide.

von Sax stood with his back to the door. Three men stood beside him deep in conversation. Prince Karl lay on the bed, his head propped up with a pillow. The patient's eyeballs fluttered behind closed lids, the sleeve of his nightshirt pulled back past his elbow. Blood streamed into a bowl from two cuts on the prince's forearm.

'What in God's name ...' Samuel exclaimed.

von Sax turned at the unexpected interruption. 'Hahnemann, who invited ...' he saw Marenzeller in the doorway. 'I thought I gave instructions to bring Hornburg. Damn you, Marenzeller, can't you follow the simplest request?'

von Sax drew himself up to his full height and stared down imperiously at Samuel. 'What we are doing is treating the prince in order to cure him. Your methods have clearly failed. The man cannot sleep. This afternoon he suffered another stroke. So much for your homeopathy, sir.'

von Sax indicated the other doctors. 'We are all agreed that the only way we can save him now is to bleed him. When we have finished, we will discuss the next step. You, sir, will not be consulted.'

57

The body of Prince Karl of Schwarzenberg lay on the table, a soiled sheet draped over the torso. Professor Clarus and Samuel Hahnemann stood with their backs to the body. Samuel wore a white mortuary gown. von Sax and a man garbed in a bloodstained smock completed the group.

Clarus read from a sheet of paper in his hand, his street clothes in stark contrast to those of his nemesis. He looked up from the paper, his eyes fixing on von Sax. 'We are agreed then. The report will show that the size of the heart was at least twice its normal size and that the walls of the right ventricle had become proportionately thin and those of the left extraordinarily thick.' von Sax nodded, beside him the fourth man also nodded. Condescendingly Clarus turned to Samuel. 'Hahnemann, are we agreed?'

Angrily Samuel nodded his head, his mouth a thin red line against the white skin.

'Then, are we further agreed, that the cause of death was a massive stroke, noting that the coronary, hepatic and splenic arteries, as well as the ascending aorta showed traces of incipient arterio-sclerosis? Clarus inclined his head to the fourth man, 'that is a true reflection of your autopsy, Beck?'

Doctor August Beck nodded. 'There is no question. But I

also want it to be noted that the condition of the body showed significant deterioration through the ingestion of alcohol.'

'Unnecessary,' Clarus interjected tersely. 'For our purposes today I think it is appropriate that the autopsy show that the cause of death was a stroke, and that is what should be reflected clearly on the medical certificate. Again, is that agreed?'

von Sax nodded. Samuel glanced at Beck, who was wiping his hands on a towel. Finally, Beck nodded, avoiding Samuel's eyes.

'Hahnemann?' Clarus asked smugly.

Samuel nodded.

'Then, could I ask each of you to sign the report so that we can release it and be done with this whole sad affair.' Clarus turned to Samuel, a supercilious sneer on his face. 'Perhaps you would sign first, Doctor Hahnemann, given that we would not need to be here today if the prince had listened to von Sax and permitted him to take the appropriate actions earlier.'

Tight-lipped Samuel picked up the quill, his eyes quickly scrolling down the familiar words. With a flourish he signed his name at the bottom.

'There, that is my duty done.' Samuel straightened his back. 'For once we are in agreement, Clarus. This has been a sad affair. But not for the want of venesection, or any other abomination. Anyone with half a mind can see the prince was doomed from the moment he was allowed to fall back into his old habits. And the blame for that must lie with the attending physician.' Samuel turned his gaze on von Sax.

'How dare you!' von Sax blazed. 'If I am not mistaken the prince asked you to be the attending physician. My position was usurped.'

'Bah!' Samuel spat back. 'I was ordered to leave his bedside five weeks ago, sir. And you were the one who gave the order. So don't lecture me now on my duties as attending physician. Unlike you, I take them very seriously.'

'Be careful of what you say in front of witnesses, Hahnemann.' Von Sax's eyes narrowed.

'Gentlemen, please,' August Beck raised his hand, 'this is most inappropriate.'

'Don't meddle, Beck,' Clarus hissed. 'Doctor von Sax, you have the sympathy of all your colleagues on the loss of your patient. It is unfortunate that Doctor Hahnemann sought to gain a certain public celebrity by treating the prince homeopathically. That it has failed will no doubt come to the attention of the medical world.'

'How dare you?' Samuel shouted, shocked at the arrogance of Clarus. 'For more than two months I have been effectively kept from the patient. Who knows what abominations von Sax and his cronies carried out in that time.'

'And your students, Doctor Hahnemann,' Clarus continued remorselessly. 'If I understand Doctor von Sax correctly, your presence became intolerable, and whilst the prince continued to exert his misguided judgement, Hornburg and Hartmann were both called into attendance.' Guilelessly Clarus turned to von Sax. 'Is that not correct, sir?'

von Sax nodded. 'Most assuredly.'

'So these immature, semi-doctors, continued to flout their positions, even though they do not yet have all the credentials they need to do so.' Clarus shook his head theatrically. 'This becomes more of a farce with each breath.' The Clinical Professor's voice suddenly became chilled. 'You chose to use the prince to support your own purposes, Hahnemann. Every doctor in Leipzig, if not all of Saxony, knows that the prince wrote to Friedrich on your behalf. Now that he is dead I wonder what our beloved King will have to say.'

58

Samuel sat slumped in his chair. Franz Hartmann stood by the door of Samuel's study, his pacing taking him from one side of the room to the other. In the armchair beside Samuel, Otto Schaefer held a sheet of paper in his hands, a bemused expression on his face.

'Samuel, surely this is not as devastating as you seem to believe?' Otto said, holding up the paper.

'No, it is worse than devastating,' Samuel said disconsolately. 'The apothecaries could hardly wait until the prince's body was in the ground before they began their petitioning of the government. That King Friedrich has effectively withdrawn his support has certainly not helped.'

'You don't know for certain ...' Franz Hartmann began.

'I don't need to see any letter from the king, Franz, to know the position was tenuous at best. If the truth be known, King Friedrich was more concerned that he should stay on the good side of his cousin than any belief in the principles of homeopathy.'

'But this is not the end of the world, Samuel.' Once again Otto Schaefer raised the piece of paper in his hand.

'Then tell me, Otto, what privileges does it give me that are not already allowed any allopathic physician.'

'Well ...'

'Read it, Otto. Please do me the honour of reminding me, out loud, how they have ridiculed me.'

'Samuel, stop this self-pity. This is not you,' Otto pleaded, fear etched into the lines around his eyes.

'Don't lecture me, Otto. Do as I have asked. Read to me where it says I can practice homeopathy the way I wish to?'

'Oh, this is ridiculous.' In two strides Hartmann was beside Otto, reaching out respectfully for the sheet of paper. Sadly Otto passed the paper over.

' ... that Doctor Hahnemann,' Hartmann began to read, 'be allowed to dispense his own medicines.' Franz Hartmann looked up from the paper and looked at Samuel, who was nodding his head slowly.

'Go on,' Samuel said, 'don't tease an old man.'

'I wasn't. I think Herr Schaefer was right, what's the point?'

Sullenly Samuel stared at the young man, his mouth shut tight.

Finally Hartmann shrugged his shoulders and returned his attention to the paper. ' ... be allowed to dispense his own medicines only when in the country where their procuration might be made difficult by the distance from the nearest town; or else in serious cases when the imminent danger does not permit the prescribing of medicines from the apothecary.'

'Enough! shouted Otto. 'This is achieving nothing, Samuel.'

'Otto, please be quiet, you haven't allowed Franz to finish, particularly the part that says I may provide medicines to the poor when the cost cannot be earned from the poor box. I think I missed one. Yes, that's right, I forgot that I'm allowed to also dispense in outlying districts where there are no apothecaries.' Samuel glared balefully at Otto. 'What they should have said was, in outlying districts where no self-respecting, profit seeking pharmacist would be foolish enough to set up practice.'

Otto lumbered to his feet, his jowls shaking in outrage. 'Samuel, I will only take so much. You have slandered my calling to my face for nearly thirty years. How many more times do you think I can accept this slur on the entire profession? There are good men out there, the pity is you have refused to accept that and tarred all of them with the same brush.'

Samuel stared up at his old friend, his mouth shut tight in a thin line of belligerence.

'Doctor Hahnemann, Herr Schaefer. Please?' Hartmann pleaded. 'What can be achieved fighting amongst yourselves?'

With his hands shaking Otto glowered at Samuel. Finally he took a deep breath and nodded slowly. 'You are right, sometimes those amongst us who should demonstrate wisdom fail to do so.' His eyes softened, but never shifted from Samuel.

A single tear escaped from the corner of Samuel's eye. 'I have had enough, Otto. If you could have seen the way Clarus humiliated me in front of von Sax and Beck.'

'I'm sure you more than held your own. You always do.'

Samuel Hahnemann shook his head. 'Not this time. Clarus slandered everything I believe in and I did nothing. I meekly accepted his ridicule.'

'The Samuel Hahnemann I know doesn't submit meekly to any man, and I refuse to believe that you have ever done so,' Otto replied softly, wary of the look of utter dejection in Samuel's eyes.

'Then you would be wrong.' He took a deep breath. 'Years ago I turned my back on practicing medicine because I abhorred the methods of treatment pursued by the doctors. Thirty years and nothing has changed. Schwarzenberg died at the hands of von Sax, just as certainly as if von Sax had driven the scalpel he'd used on his arm directly into the prince's heart.'

'So you intend to give up?' Otto asked quietly, 'give up when half the country is finally starting to take notice.' Schaefer looked across at young Hartmann. 'It is not only your disciples who you are abandoning, Samuel. What of your patients? Men like Goethe, his literary friends and other influential people in the arts have come out in the journals and supported your principles. Tell me, do you propose to desert them too?'

'Of course not, but ...'

'There can be no but, Samuel,' Otto said firmly. 'You started this, you must finish it. Otherwise what faith can men like Franz have in you or homeopathy?'

Samuel slumped further into his chair, his head dropping into his hands. 'Otto, I am so tired of this, so tired.' He lifted his face to peer up at Schaefer, tears pricking at the corners of his eyes. 'Don't you understand? I don't know if I have the strength to fight any further.'

Samuel turned his blurred gaze on Franz Hartmann, who had returned to his post by the door. Tears streamed down the young doctor's face. Hartmann brushed his cheeks, smearing the flow. 'Herr Schaefer is right, Doctor Hahnemann,' Hartmann mumbled through his tears. If the fight has gone from you, what hope is there for the rest of us?'

Wrenching the door open, Franz Hartmann stumbled into the passageway and fled the house.

59

Franz Hartmann heard the knock on the door, resolving that whoever it was would tire of their enquiry and leave. He turned his attention to the glowing coals in the small fire in his hearth. The miserable winter had been long and hard on everyone.

Once more his ears pricked to the knocking on his door. 'Leave me alone,' he muttered to himself. The pounding continued booming into his rooms.

'All right. All right. I'm coming. Leave the door be.'

He crossed to the door and opened it. Three men waited. Franz Hartmann's heart skipped a beat. Professor Clarus stood in front of two university marshalls whose faces were set with determination, their ceremonial robes of office strangely intimidating.

'Ah, young Hartmann, you are at home. Your landlord thought he'd seen you come in.' Clarus smiled, his attempt at being disarming only managing to appear evil.

'Yes, I was, er, lost in my studies,' Hartmann said grimly. 'Professor, I'm not accustomed to receiving such esteemed visitors to my humble lodgings. How can I help you?'

Clarus held the eye of the young man for a moment longer than was necessary and then turned to the taller of the two beadles. He held out his hand. The official took a scroll from inside his robe and passed it to the Clinical Professor.'

Clarus unrolled the scroll and then sought the young student's eyes. 'The university has charged me with the most onerous task.' He looked down at the scroll and then back at Hartmann. 'The High Court of the University has decreed that no student of the university should be entitled to practice until such a time as they have satisfied all the examinations required by the university.' Clarus paused again, his eyes seeking the words on the page in his hand. 'Further, the High Court has decreed that no student of the university shall be entitled to practice homeopathy until such a time as they have satisfied the court that they are proficient in all aspects of medical training.' Clarus stopped reading, a sly smile appearing on his lips. 'We already have proof, Herr Hartmann, that you have been seeing patients. I am sure you will not deny the conviction against you in the university's records.'

Franz Hartmann was too stunned at what was unfolding to defend himself.

'No, we didn't believe you would try to protest your innocence on that matter, given your appeal to the university to hear your *viva voce*. 'There is one further decree that the High Court has issued, which I counsel you to attend to wisely.'

Hartmann raised his eyebrows, his voice still forsaking him.

'From this point forward, and following the court action taken by the Town Council and the State against Samuel Hahnemann, the university has decreed that no student should be in possession of any homeopathic medicines for any purpose whatsoever. Thereby I am instructed by the High Court to confiscate any such medicines that you may have in your rooms or on your person.'

'You wouldn't dare ...' Franz Hartmann spluttered.

Arrogantly Clarus held out the decree for the young student to take. 'If you doubt me, sir, read it for yourself.' He turned to the officials standing behind him. 'If you please.' He held out his arm inviting them to enter.

'What are you doing?' Hartmann cried out.

'I have the permission and authority of the university to search your rooms if you don't cooperate.'

'Herr Schaefer, thank God that I found you in.' Franz Hartmann stood at the foot of the stairs as the portly apothecary padded down from his room.

'Franz, what is it, what could be so important to steal a man's afternoon nap? The poor innkeeper's wife was most distressed at your determination to wake me.'

'I am sorry, Herr Schaefer, I apologise for my impertinence but I had to seek advice from someone. You were the only person I felt I would be able to trust.'

'Advice for what? My goodness what has happened, you are certainly distraught. Come, let us find a seat in the dining room.' Otto took the young man's elbow and led him through to the empty dining room. 'By the way, before I forget, Johann Stapf will be arriving shortly. He wrote to say that he would be visiting Leipzig and asked if I would be here. Now, what can I give you advice on?'

'I'm at a complete loss, sir. I've just had Clarus and his musclemen... '

'Clarus and his musclemen? ... I'm not sure I understand.'

'The beadles, his so-called ceremonial marshals.'

'All right,' Otto nodded, 'to do what?'

'The university High Court has decreed that no student can practice medicine until they are qualified.'

'That seems eminently sensible to me. Otherwise we could have anyone out there ...'

'I know, I know, but some of us ... Hornburg and I have been practicing homeopathy because people have pleaded with us to treat them.'

'Pleaded with you?'

'Yes! Patients know it works, so as soon as they hear that someone has treated somebody they clamour at our door.'

'I am only too aware of the spreading reputation of homeopathy but I had no idea that patients would harass students;

fully qualified doctors like Samuel and Johann Stapf, I can understand.'

Hartmann nodded. 'Well they have. Christian and I have been able to earn money to help pay for our studies.'

'And now you say it is banned, along with the practicing of any discipline by students.'

Again Hartmann nodded.

'So how will this affect your *viva voce*?'

'I have no idea, Herr Schaefer, but please let me finish.'

'There is more to this astonishing story?' Otto asked wide-eyed.

'Most definitely. Clarus had also been given authority to search my rooms for any homeopathic remedies I was keeping.'

'To search ... and did they find what they were looking for?'

'Of course, I never denied having them. Why should I, there is nothing illegal about it.'

'Obviously the university thinks otherwise. So what did they do? Confiscate the remedies?'

Hartmann nodded, a perplexed look on his face. 'Yes, they did. Then they carried them away in a bizarre ceremony, the phials carried high.'

'This is the most strange behaviour.'

'Herr Schaefer, you've only heard the half of it. I followed them from my lodgings. Clarus led them to St Paul's, to the church yard where the beadles proceeded to bury them in the ground.'

A knock on the door interrupted the two men. Johann Stapf entered without waiting for an invitation. He shook Otto Schaefer warmly by the hand then turned to Hartmann. 'Franz, I'm pleased you're here.' Stapf reached into the inside of his overcoat and extracted a copy of the *Leipziger Zeitung*. He laid the paper down on the table and turned to an inside page. 'I fear that the persecution of Samuel has really begun in earnest. This time thirteen of Leipzig's supposed finest, including the indefatigable Professor Clarus, have launched a scathing attack on his treatments. I truly fear that this might finally tip Samuel over the edge.'

60

'Gentlemen, he is not at home. He said he had a lecture at the university.' Caroline led Otto Schaefer into her father's study.. 'Stapf and Hartmann followed the portly apothecary.

'What mood was he in when he left?' Stapf asked of Caroline's back.

The young woman spoke over her shoulder. 'When he finished his morning's surgery he ate some lunch and then returned to his study to collect his things. He seemed no different to yesterday or the day before. He doesn't speak very much at the lunch table.' Caroline shook her head. 'I'm not sure how to answer. Since the court ruling he has been withdrawn,'

'No more so than before though, you would say?' Otto Schaefer asked.

Again Caroline shook her head. 'Should he be?'

Abruptly Otto Schaefer stopped, his eye caught by something on Samuel's desk. He crossed the room and picked up the paper spread open on the leather inlay. 'Did your father make any comment about this Caroline?' Otto held up the copy of the *Leipziger Zeitung*.

Caroline shook her head. 'No, as I said, he hardly spoke at lunch. Uncle Otto, please, you are frightening me. What is happening?'

'A group of doctors have attacked your father about his

methods of treatment. We were worried that he might have reacted badly to it.'

'Is that the article?'

Otto nodded and handed the paper to Caroline. 'I'm going to the university,' he said. 'I want to talk to Samuel about his reply.'

'His reply. What reply?' asked Johann Stapf.

'The one he must write to refute these fools.'

'But what good will that do?' Hartmann joined in.

'It will prove that he hasn't given up,' Otto said and kissed Caroline on the cheek, oblivious to the stunned look on her face.

'Johann, please explain to me again about the article Samuel wrote which triggered this response.' Otto tapped the paper on his knee.

Stapf and Otto Schaefer sat opposite each other in the carriage. Hartmann lounged next to Stapf, his attention taken by something in the Burgstrasse.

Stapf leant forward, his hands on his knees, his body swaying gently with the carriage. 'Samuel identified an outbreak of an eruptive fever as purpura miliaris and not scarlet fever, which appeared to be the consensus of most doctors.'

'So the treatment would have been different?'

'That's right, aconite instead of belladonna. And that was Samuel's motive for writing the article. He saw it as a service not only to the other doctors but to the people of Leipzig.' Stapf smiled grimly. 'In his usual style he couldn't resist firing a salvo across the bows of the Town Council and the doctors.'

Otto rolled his eyes.

Johann Stapf noted the reaction. 'Even when he is down he still seems to come up with a good line. Don't ask me to quote it verbatim Otto, but it was something about feeling bound to show his deep veneration to the people of Leipzig, as it was now impossible to serve them actively.'

Otto smiled, recalling to his mind a picture of the young Samuel Hahnemann he'd met in his pharmacy in Molschleben and how the fire had burned in his eyes.

'Otto ...?'

'Sorry, Johann, I was just thinking about Samuel, how the man's passion has driven him.'

Johann Stapf nodded. 'We all remember. Oh, for goodness sake,' he slapped his hand on his knee, 'we're talking as if the fire is extinguished. And I don't believe that. Samuel is far too strong.' Stapf pointed at the paper in Otto's hand. 'Can you believe that those thirteen doctors have denounced Samuel for supposedly making the claim that he discovered belladonna.'

'Doctor Hahnemann would never claim anything so foolish,' Franz Hartmann cried. 'Belladonna has been used for centuries.'

Stapf grinned at his young friend and then returned his attention to Otto. 'As any half-smart student knows. Of course, what Samuel discovered was that belladonna would cure scarlet fever.' He shook his head. 'If only these fools would bother to read the *Organon*, if only they would dare to know.'

Stapf and Hartmann both recognised the two professors walking across the courtyard and nodded. The two members of the medical faculty dropped their heads and swept past without acknowledgment. Stapf raised an eyebrow at his younger colleague, who shrugged disconsolately.

'That is the way it has been for months,' Hartmann said. 'Professor Clarus has whipped up something close to loathing among the faculty. The younger students tell me they daren't risk discussing homeopathy openly for fear of being ostracised by the other professors.'

'This is medieval,' Otto Schaefer cut in. 'Haven't the other professors any spirit?'

'Don't forget that Clarus can act as judge and prosecutor simply by virtue of his position. There are not many who are prepared to stand up to him.'

'They do his bidding without question,' Hartmann added. 'It is sickening to watch them fawn over him.'

'What of Rosenmüller?' Otto asked.

Hartmann replied, 'I suspect the politics of it are even too great for the Dean.'

A third professor hurried past the group, his face averted. As they entered the large portal that heralded the medical building on the edge of the courtyard, Otto looked over his shoulder. Except for the fleeing professor it was empty. 'The university is surprisingly quiet, Franz. Is this normal for a Saturday afternoon?'

'No. I must admit there is a very sombre mood hanging over the old place. Wouldn't you agree, Johann?'

Stapf nodded. 'Maybe it's the whiff of persecution that has pervaded the place. The faculty members are too guilty to show their heads and the students prefer the sanctuary of their rooms or the library to conduct their reading.' He looked down the wide corridor, the flagged stone under foot resounded with hollow slaps as they walked. 'Which lecture room does Samuel use, Franz? Still the same one?'

'I don't think he has moved once, not since he first came here nine years ago.'

Is it nine years since that amazing dissertation?' Otto shook his head.

'I was there,' Stapf said. 'It was a year before my bachelor's examination. He made not one mention of homeopathy and gave no indication of the furore that was to follow, yet I was mesmerised. I was compelled to attend his first lecture.'

'I had planned to, but other matters kept me away.' Otto smiled sadly at the memory of his son.

Two men approached from the other end of the corridor. One wore an academic gown, the other, a large bear of a man, was wearing a thick top-coat over his street clothes. As they came closer Otto recognised Albert Wagner.

Otto lifted his hand to his tricorn. 'Alb ...' he began.

The rest of his words were lost as Wagner stormed past, his eyes never wavering from the floor. Stunned, Otto turned and watched the back of the apothecary as he headed for the front door. With a surprised shake of his head Otto resumed walking, reaching the corner without a word.

'Here is the lecture room, gentlemen,' Hartmann said.

'Should we wait out here until he is finished?' he inquired of his companions. The soft drone of a voice vibrated through the timber.

'I'm sure Samuel won't mind if we enter quietly,' Otto said, still unsettled by the appearance of Wagner. He brightened when he saw the questioning faces of his two colleagues. Otto smiled, 'I must admit, after all these years I am still a little intrigued to see the theatre of his performances again.'

Stapf joined in with a soft smile, also trying to lighten the sullenness of their encounter in the corridor. 'I agree. It is time that I also gave serious thought to improving my knowledge and returning to some selective study. The sanctity of the lecture room has been missing from my life. Perhaps the smell and the sound of it will get me inspired.'

Otto Schaefer knocked gently on the door and opened it. With mock gravity he stood back as his two younger friends entered the room. A sharp intake of breath from Stapf made Otto twist his head and peer into the room.

Samuel stood in front of the small table, the *Organon* resplendent against the timber, several sheets of white parchment and a quill beside it. The good doctor waved his hands dramatically as he spoke in the way that Otto had remembered so fondly. Samuel paused, wanting his point to sink in. Then he resumed again, his voice flowing across the lecture theatre.

Otto's heart was thudding in his chest as he turned to look at the rest of the room.

The first row of seats was empty.

His gaze moved onto the second.

The second row was as bare of students as the first.

His eyes flicked to the next. Empty. Then the next.

Frantically Otto looked to the back of the large room, his eyes searching every row, every corner.

Finally he gave up and turned back to look at his two colleagues. Their faces were drained, as he knew his own would be. Forlornly he looked back to the room knowing that no amount of searching could change the fact that there was not another soul there.

61

Gently Otto touched his friend's elbow. Samuel Hahnemann stopped speaking, his head falling forward to his chest.

'Samuel, my old friend,' Otto said softly. He waited for a response but none came. 'Why don't you allow us to take you home? Perhaps we could enjoy one of your fine pilseners.'

'Doctor Hahnemann ...' Franz Hartmann began, only to fall silent at a shake of Johann Stapf's head.

Samuel's shoulders shook.

'Samuel, please, you are surely in shock,' Otto said. 'There is no-one here, Samuel. Do you understand me? There is no-one in the lecture room to hear your wise words.' Otto gently wrapped his arm around his old friend's shoulder. 'Come, my friend, let us go home.'

Samuel Hahnemann lifted his head and looked out over the empty rows of seats. He made no attempt to acknowledge that he had heard or understood Otto's words.

'Samuel, please tell me you understand me? There is no-one here to listen.' Otto looked over Samuel's head at Johann Stapf, who was standing on the other side of their friend. Franz Hartmann moved to the small table and stared down at the pieces of paper.

Otto squeezed his friend's arm. 'Samuel, look at me. Do you

hear me? There is no-one here.'

Samuel took a deep breath and looked into Otto's eyes. 'I know, Otto. There has not been anyone for weeks.' He let out a sigh and closed his eyes. When he opened them a tear leaked from the corner. 'The students are too frightened to come. Clarus has won. He has threatened to fail anyone who attends my lectures.'

'Herr Schaefer, I think you should read this.' Franz Hartmann tugged at the apothecary's sleeve. 'Johann, you also, this paper is ...'

'Is an advice from the apothecaries,' Samuel interjected quietly, 'that they intend to make further representation to the High Court.'

'Further representation for what?' stammered Johann Stapf, grateful that his mentor seemed to have shaken off any sign of madness.

Samuel remained silent, appearing not to have heard the question.

'Samuel! Representation to do what?' Otto asked anxiously.

A tear ran down his friend's cheek but no more words were uttered.

'Look,' Hartmann proffered the paper in his hand. 'It is signed by Albert Wagner on behalf of the apothecaries.'

Unconsciously Otto turned his head to the door and the corridor beyond where he had been rebuffed by the man minutes before.

'It is a letter to Doctor Hahnemann,' young Hartmann continued, 'telling him that the apothecaries have petitioned the High Court to have him forcibly removed from the city.'

'To have him forcibly removed? Why?' Johann Stapf cried out in pain.

'They have written to the court saying that they believe Doctor Hahnemann will abuse the privileges granted him to dispense his medicines.'

'Privileges?' an outraged Otto Schaefer said. 'His so-called privileges aren't worth the paper they're written on.' He turned to Hartmann, holding out his hand. 'May I.'

Hartmann handed the paper to Otto Schaefer. Otto peered at Wagner's signature at the bottom. He imagined the arrogant apothecary taking great delight in hand delivering this final blow.

Meanwhile Hartmann picked up the second piece of paper. 'It would seem that Doctor Hahnemann was preparing for one final battle when he received that.'

Distracted, Schaefer looked up. 'What? What do you mean, Franz?'

'Obviously Doctor Hahnemann was one step ahead of us. He must have been working on his reply to the thirteen doctors.' Hartmann handed the paper to Otto Schaefer who looked at the first few lines. He gazed up at Johann Stapf and then at his old friend before returning to the paper.

Otto Schaefer read aloud. 'Just look now, there stand thirteen gentlemen — so-called colleagues of mine in this town — who are struggling hard to show the readers that they envy my reputation (such as it is), my discoveries, my writings (which they will not read) and my cures, which, by the grace of God, I have successfully effected on patients... '

Otto turned the page over in his hand, searching the other side. He raised an eyebrow and looked at his old friend, who was staring blindly at the wall at the back of the room. 'That's where it ends.'

Samuel blinked and turned to his friend. 'No, Otto, that's not where it ends. I will never give in. You of all people should know that.' A tear escaped and ran down his cheek. 'But I am tired. I am so tired.' He smiled a distant smile at his friend, then shifted his gaze to embrace Johann Stapf and Franz Hartmann.

'I'm truly sorry. For the moment, I am too tired to continue this fight. There are too many against me.'

Postscript

On the 21st of February, 1821, common sense prevailed and the call by the apothecaries to have Samuel forcibly removed from Leipzig was rejected by the High Court. But their appeal did not go completely unrewarded. In its judgement, the court added a codicil that reinforced the power of the apothecaries. 'Although the matters must remain as determined by the Royal judgement, the apothecaries should report any cases of misuse occurring.'

Not prepared to let this injustice lie, Samuel's friends once more waded into the fray. Doctor Volkmann, the Town Clerk of Leipzig, entered a protest in the Appeal Court of Dresden against the treatment of Samuel by the doctors and apothecaries. Joining Volkmann in the protest were forty of Leipzig's finest citizens. The Appeal Court upheld the protest and ruled that Hahnemann had every right to remain in Leipzig and should not be prey to the persecution of the apothecaries. Unfortunately this judgement did not have the power to overturn the royal decree effectively preventing Samuel from dispensing medicines, and thereby practicing homeopathy.

In the meantime Samuel had resolved that he would leave Leipzig. At the age of 66 he took his family and moved to Köthen. There, Grand Duke Ferdinand, ruler of the principality, offered

Samuel both the rights to practice homeopathy and the right to dispense his own remedies. For the next nine years he practiced his craft in relative peace and seclusion, remaining in contact with his friends through regular letters. Then, in 1830, his beloved Elise passed away at the age of 67.

Samuel was seventy-five, well past the age most men and women were expected to live, but still far from finished in his fight to establish homeopathy.

In 1831 cholera reached epidemic proportions throughout Western Europe. Samuel Hahnemann had already predicted that conventional treatment of cholera would be ineffective.

The medical profession and the public were thrown into a state of panic. Thousands died. Villages took the law into their own hands, threatening to kill any strangers who came to their town who might carry the plague. Samuel wrote four essays on the treatment of cholera, which were published widely. Unfortunately very few allopathic doctors followed his directions even though reports from across Europe showed that the death rate amongst patients being treated with conventional medicines exceeded 50 percent while those being treated homeopathically was as low as 2 percent.

Once again the medical fraternity and the apothecaries united against Samuel. Pressure was brought to bear and a royal decree was issued, withdrawing the rights of homeopaths to prepare or dispense their own remedies.

It is of little comfort that, years later, Samuel was proven right.

In his published articles he had identified that the disease was spread by a small, invisible living organism, a concept which was significantly ahead of its time. Sixty-seven years later, just before the turn of the 20th century, Samuel's predictions were validated when the nature and existence of the cholera bacterium was isolated.

Samuel finally moved to Paris where he remarried and lived happily with his new wife until his death in 1843.

He was 88 years old.

His fellow collaborators, who remained to continue the fight in Saxony, were not all so fortunate.

Samuel's devoted disciple, Karl Franz, was persecuted by Professor Clarus following the death from tuberculosis of one of the young doctor's female patients. Franz was forced to retire and pay the costs of the court, even though the charges were never substantiated.

Christian Hornburg, one of Samuel's original team of provers, suffered even greater persecution under the hands of Clarus. Hornburg achieved stunning success in the treatment of his patients, even while still a student. Unfortunately he made an enemy of Clarus and other members of the faculty. Clarus twice arranged for Christian to fail his examinations. Instead of providing a caution, these actions inflamed Hornburg, who took to abusing and ridiculing allopathic doctors. He became bolder and more obnoxious, further enraging the establishment and causing his rejection by every university he approached to take his bachelor's examination. The final blow came in 1831 when Clarus instituted a criminal investigation into the death of a woman, accusing Hornburg of hastening the woman's death by unsuitable measures. He was convicted and sentenced to two months imprisonment, but died, at the age of 41, before he could be sent to prison.

Franz Hartmann did go to Dresden and passed the required state examination. In 1821 he practiced for the first time in a little town called Zschopau. Due to the poverty of the area, his rising fame didn't translate into money and he was required to move to Leipzig. Like his mentor he turned to literary work and was the author of many influential treatises on homeopathy. He also published a work that he hoped would make the principles of homeopathy more accessible to the physicians of the old school. Ironically this brought Hartmann into conflict with his old mentor, who rejected any suggestion of conciliating the allopaths. Despite this, Hartmann continued to revere his master and provided some of the most insightful and affectionate descriptions of Samuel Hahnemann ever recorded. Franz Hartmann died at the age of 57, having struggled for many years as an invalid.

Over the years Johann Stapf became Samuel Hahnemann's closest confidante and friend. Right up until Samuel's death he maintained a lively correspondence. Stapf became an increasingly sought-after physician, even being called to London in 1835 to treat the Queen of England. Stapf was also a prolific writer and penned numerous articles and dissertations on every possible question of homeopathy. Throughout his life he remained a true disciple of Samuel and a zealous defender of homeopathy. Johann Stapf died in 1860 at the age of 71.

And what of Otto Schaefer? I think I would have liked Otto had he ever existed in any place other than my imagination. Hopefully Otto went to Heaven, rather than in the place his fellow fictional apothecary, Albert Wagner, no doubt finished up.

Today, homeopathy thrives in many countries around the world.

It is the backbone of the Indian medical system, where homeopathic doctors treat millions of patients every week. In England, France and Germany, and other parts of Europe, homeopathy thrives, often with royal patronage. In the US, homeopathy has had a rebirth and is slowly assuming the strength it held in that country in the 19th and early 20th centuries.

However, even now, more than 250 years after the birth of Samuel Hahnemann, the master no doubt turns in his grave each night knowing that, in many countries, the modern day apothecaries are still persecuting his philosophy.